Change Your Mind Change Your Weight

by Dr. Raeleen D'Agostino Mautner

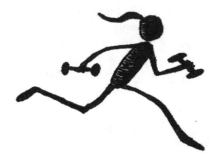

RONIN

BERKELEY, CA

Change Your Mind Change Your Weight
ISBN: 1-57951-060-4
Copyright © 2002 by Ronin Publishing, Inc.

Published by
RONIN Publishing, Inc.
PO Box 22900
Oakland, CA 94609
roninpub.com

Credits:

Editor:	Beverly A. Potter
	docpotter.com
Cover Design:	Brian Groppe
Interior Design:	Beverly A. Potter
Illustrations:	Casey Mautner
Fonts:	Cutout
	Gouty Old Style
	Pompeia Inline
	Quetzalcoat
	Times

Distributed to the trade by Publishers Group West
Printed in the United States of America by Bertelsmann

Library of Congress Card Number: 2002111534

Acknowledgements

I THANK MY FAMILY AND FRIENDS, whose patience and support have been invaluable to me. I also thank the following very special people who believed in and supported the message of this book and who contributed their valuable time and expertise to help make it a success.

A special note of gratitude goes to Docpotter, my publisher at Ronin Publishing, who was always available to answer questions, share information, and involve me in the entire book-making process.

I am in awe of Dr. Albert Ellis—the originator of the ABCDE paradigm of Rational Emotive Behavior Therapy and Cognitive Behavior Therapy. Dr Ellis changed the face of psychotherapy and made psychological well-being a possibility for all of us. I appreciatively draw upon his ABCDE model. I've also drawn upon the "learned optimism" approach of the distinguished Dr. Martin E.P. Seligman to create a solid, cognitive restructuring approach for *Change Your Mind, Change Your Weight*.

I am so pleased that Brad Schoenfeld, an expert in the field of fitness, contributed the Foreword to this book. As president of Global Fitness Services and best selling author of two wonderful fitness books, Mr. Schoenfeld has helped spread the word to millions of Americans—especially women—about the importance of lifting weights for overall fitness. His enthusiasm and sincerity are contagious.

Last but not least, I thank my daughter Casey Mautner for her insightful work in designing the illustrations.

About Dr. Mautner

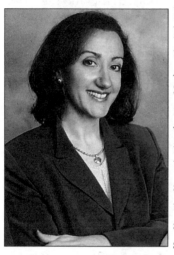

RAELEEN D'AGOSTINO MAUTNER is an assistant professor of Psychology at Albertus Magnus College. She earned her doctorate in Educational Psychology with an emphasis on Cognitive Psychology from the University of Connecticut and has worked as an international research consultant, as well as a behavioral consultant for a hospital-based weight-loss program. Dr. Mautner is the author of *Living la Dolce Vita: Bring the Passion, Laughter and Serenity of Italy into Your Daily Life*, which is a Mediterranean approach to mental and physical well-being. Please visit her site at www.MindLifeSolutions.com

A well written, exceptionally clear book that will help many people with their weight reduction problems. Includes some of the main findings of Rational Emotive Behavior Therapy and Cognitive Behavior Therapy accurately and simply stated for willing readers.

–Albert Ellis, Ph.D.
President, Albert Ellis Institute, NYC
author of
A Guide to Rational Living

Table
of Contents

Foreword

by Brad Schoenfeld

LOSING WEIGHT IS BIG BUSINESS. From diet books to nutritional supplements to magic creams and beyond, the weight loss industry generates billions of dollars a year in revenues. And with the public's seemingly unending appetite (no pun intended!) for novel ways to burn fat, new products are being introduced on an almost daily basis.

But in spite of all the hype, the solution to long-term weight management is fairly straightforward: you need to budget calories. This follows the laws of thermodynamics: if you take in fewer calories than you expend you'll lose weight; if you take in more calories than you expend you'll gain weight. Sounds simple, right? It is. Unfortunately, though, following this formula is not as easy as it seems.

The sad fact is that America is getting fatter and fatter each year. With all of our amazing advances in nutritional science, about 2/3 of the population remains overweight and more than 20 percent are considered clinically obese. Moreover, the statistics of those who attempt to diet are equally alarming: approximately 90 percent regain their previous weight within a year's time.

The primary reason why diets fail to produce lasting results is because they are short-term solutions to a long-term problem and don't adequately address the change in lifestyle that is necessary to sustain ongoing weight management. Sure, anyone can lose weight by following a pre-fabricated diet that reduces calories below baseline levels. But once you've slimmed down, the question then becomes "what's next?"

I'm happy to say that *Change Your Mind, Change Your Weight* is the book to tell you "what's next." It addresses the importance of developing a sound nutritional strategy and offers a sensible plan of action for combating the battle of the bulge. But unlike most diet books, it doesn't advocate a specific dietary program for rapid weight loss. Rather, it teaches you how to approach eating from a cognitive perspective. Once you develop the proper nutritional mindset, adhering to a long-term dietary regimen becomes second nature.

Dr. Mautner has done an excellent job of putting this book together. She doesn't pull any punches and tackles a complex subject in a very forthright manner. In effect, she acts as your own personal weight loss coach, helping you conquer the psychological aspects of losing weight. She delivers practical advice on the realities of weight loss and provides solid guidance on how to deal with the many hurdles that you will inevitably face in your quest to get lean.

It is particularly refreshing to see that Dr. Mautner recommends dedicated exercise as an integral part of a weight loss program. Studies consistently show that those who combine exercise with diet are more successful in losing weight over the long haul. Yet all too often, this essential component is completely neglected by today's "diet gurus."

As far as exercise specifics, make sure to lift weights. While cardiovascular training certainly helps to expedite fat loss, lifting weights is the most important activity you can perform. Not only does it produce a firm, shapely physique, but it also helps to reduce bodyfat. You see, muscle is metabolically active tissue. For each pound of muscle that you gain, your body burns approximately 50 calories a day at rest. Hence, by adding several pounds of lean muscle to your physique, you turn your body into a fat burning machine that works 'round the clock to fight flab. Bottom line: You must work out—if not, your chances of maintaining a lean body are tenuous at best.

In sum, I urge you to embrace the principles outlined in this book. It is a solid, well-written, and well-researched guide to losing weight and, more importantly, keeping it off permanently. By combining proper exercise and nutrition with the right mental approach, your ultimate success in maintaining a healthy, fit body is all but guaranteed. -Stay Fit!

—Brad Schoenfeld, CSCS

author of

Look Great Naked &

Sculpting Her Body Perfect

www.lookgreatnaked.com

Introduction

THE BOOK YOU ARE ABOUT TO READ will strike you as refreshingly candid or painfully honest, depending on your frame of mind. Your frame of mind, incidentally, has a huge influence on weight-loss and so I thought it only fitting to make it the focus of this book. You are about to become an expert on getting your thoughts and emotions to work to your advantage. *Change Your Mind, Change Your Weight* tells what it takes to reach the healthy, sensible weight that your body and mind deserve—no holds barred.

The research has long established that being overweight has negative physical and psychological ramifications. What you may not have known is that what goes on in your head has a powerful influence on what goes on with your weight. If you remember only one thing from this book let it be this: The key to weight loss success lies in the way you *think*, and *what you tell yourself* when times get rough.

> The key to weight loss success lies in the way you *think*.

What we say to ourselves when we encounter setbacks determines what happens in the critical

Reacting to setbacks with rational optimism lays the foundation for success.

moments that follow. The key is to oversome obstacles by retaining a positive perspective. Reacting negatively leads to a state of psychological helplessness. This mental "inertia" has a demoralizing effect on goal-oriented efforts and leads to anxiety and depression. Learning to react to setbacks with rational optimism—remaining positive while maintaining a strong foothold in reality—lays the foundation for success. When we can prove to ourselves that setbacks are just temporary and surmountable, they lose the power to unravel us. *There is something you can do.* And I am about to show you how to do it. Now let's get moving!

1
IT'S ALL
ATTITUDE

TTITUDE HAS A MORE POWERFUL EFFECT on weight-loss than any other factor. The process of shedding pounds is no different from anything else in life—we take a few steps forward and occasionally slide backward. That's only natural. Along the way, we automatically—often subconsciously—make judgments about the reasons for our victories and losses. If you go on a beet-and-cabbage diet on Monday and then dive into a half-gallon of ice-cream for breakfast on Tuesday, of course you will not lose weight. Moreover, you will probably conclude that diets don't work. However illogical our beliefs and conclusions may be, they will determine whether we reach our goals or not. If your attitude towards weight-loss plans is that they don't work, why would you bother starting over again?

Fortunately, there is an effective way to render self-defeating thoughts powerless. Determine your *current* attitude towards weight-loss, and then shape that attitude to your advantage. The following quiz will give help you assess your attitude about losing weight.

What is Your Weight-Loss Attitude?

Instructions: Think of how you feel about trying to lose weight as you read and respond to each item below. Using a scale from 1 to 5, with 1 being "rarely true" and 5 being "usually true," rate how true the item is for you. Don't spend too much time deliberating over each item; just choose the first rating that comes to mind.

Rarely true 1- 2 - 3 - 4 - 5 Usually true

___1. When I go off my diet, I also stop exercising.
___2. If I skip exercise I can't get back into it.
___3. I'll never lose weight because I'm lazy.
___4. When my life, goes wrong I drop my fitness plans.
___5. I've tried losing weight many times; nothing works.
___6. Losing weight is just too hard for me.
___7. I can't lose weight because I lack willpower.
___8. My parents were heavy, and that's my fate, too.
___9. Everyone seems able to loose weight but me.
___10. Exercise programs are basically useless.
___11. Once I start eating I can't stop.
___12. I'm addicted to the wrong foods.

Scoring:

12–24 **Weight-Loss Optimist:** Your rational optimism will help you achieve your weight-loss goals. Maintain your positive views of your ability to stick to your program and you will achieve your desired weight.

25–48 **Weight-Loss Hopeful:** You are generally optimistic about being able to lose weight. Bolster your positive thinking to give yourself a boost in overcoming the difficulties of losing weight.

49–60 **Weight-Loss Pessimist:** Your lack of confidence in your ability to loss weight underminds your success. Change the way you think to curb your defeatist attitude and losing weight will become easier.

Those who take an optimistic perspective towards losing weight have more energy and determination to reach their goals than do their negative-thinking counterparts. Optimists don't waste time when something they attempt doesn't work. Instead they turn setbacks into lessons, and then into solutions. You can't fail with a wining attitude like that!

Negative thinking snowballs. It is easy to get discouraged about losing

> Optimists turn setbacks into lessons.

weight and to see setbacks as more important than they are. When you get trapped in pessimistic thinking your mind tries to convince you that a slip-up is a sign of your incompetence. You think you are doomed to repeat your mistake or that you are a failure in general because you overate today. Negative thinking feeds upon itself, and berating ourselves makes us feel hopeless and unmotivated.

Change Your Attitude!

DON'T GET DISCOURAGED. There is a way out! A little attitude adjustment here and there will get you back up and running to the finish line. If you change your style of thinking you will be able to wipe out the self-defeating thoughts that stand between you and your weight-loss goals.

You must train yourself to catch these thoughts as they occur. Berating ourselves makes us feel hopeless and unmotivated. If you scored low in weight-loss optimism, you probably interpret normal setbacks as more catastrophic than they really are. Your mind tries to convince you that a slip-up is a sign of your incompetence, and that you are doomed to failure—so why bother trying? It's never too late to reverse insidious pessimistic thinking habits. To do so you must be willing to roll up your sleeves and work hard.

The more you challenge your self-defeating thoughts, the less likely they are to return. By following the techniques in this book you have a head start in becoming a full-fledged weight-loss optimist, and permanently training your mind to turn setbacks into successes.

Attribution is Key

PSYCHOLOGIST BERNARD WEINER found that the difference between achievers and non-achievers doesn't depend on the *number* of failures or successes a person has, but rather on the *conclusions* one draws about why those successes and failures happened. He called this Attribution Theory.

Pessimism

IN GENERAL, IF A PERSON "ATTRIBUTES" FAILURE to a personal defect—like incompetence—and explains success as a stroke of luck, then he is reasoning like a pessimist. Pessimistic thinking is wrought with a sense of helplessness. Helplessness is the emotional inertia we feel when we are depressed. We feel like nothing we do will make a difference, so why bother? When we are in this sort of emotional state we perceive the smallest obstacles as insurmountable hurdles. Such a mindset is not only counterproductive when trying to lose weight—it is disastrous! A defeatist attitude saps energy and destroys motivation to stick with a weight-loss program.

> Pessimistic thinking engenders feelings of helplessness.

Optimism

AN OPTIMISTIC ATTITUDE generates hope and persistence—which, coincidentally, are the ingredients required to make permanent weight-loss changes! This positive perspective must take *reality* into account for it to work. Ignoring difficulties doesn't make them disappear—focusing on solutions does.

> Optimistic thinking generates hope and persistence.

The Weight-Loss Maize

HAVE YOU NOTICED that the moment you finally make the decision to lose weight everyone from your long-lost aunt to your neighbor's dog jumps out of the woodwork to tell you what to do—or to let you know how *they* did it?   Diet and exercise books propel themselves into your hands from bookstore shelves, where, ironically you can digest them along with a latte' and croissant.   If you manage to cut through the contradictory advice, and the staggering hodgepodge of weight-loss literature, you will notice that weight-loss information generally falls into two categories: Short-term weight-loss fads, and long-term weight-loss approaches that emphasize developing new life-style habits.

Weight Loss Fads

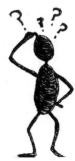

FADS INCLUDE NONSENSICAL DIETS and rigorous workout programs that Hercules himself would have had trouble committing to. Diets that primarily emphasize one type of food or beverage, fit this category.   Heart-stopping exercise regimes belong to this approach as well. Our quest for a magic pill that promises to save us from a continued string of weight-loss attempts and failures attracts us to these extremes. These programs are neither practical nor safe for the long haul. Deep down you know there is no easy way out.

Developing New Habits

LIFESTYLE-ORIENTED PROGRAMS WORK. Sensible, research-based programs, which are endorsed by respected experts and health associations are the reliable approach. Once you form a daily habit of simple clean eating and moderate activity, you *will* lose weight—and feel pretty good in the process.

The drawback to the sensible approach is that results are slow, the techniques are non-dramatic, and we get bored. We become impatient and find it hard to stick with a program long enough to reap the benefits.

Even if you have lost some weight using one approach or the other, over time your motivation probably dwindled, and the lost pounds were quickly regained. You are not alone in your frustration! You may have mastered the nutritional and exercise fundamentals to a tee, yet still haven't attained your fitness goals. Why? Because in addition to learning to eat and exercise properly, there is one more skill you need—mastering your mind! A re-trained *attitude* is the only map that can get you out of the confusing forest of "dietville" once and for all.

> To achieve weight-loss goals you must eat properly, exercise regularly —and master your mind!

Change Your Mind

WEIGHT LOSS THROUGH MENTAL SELF-MASTERY is the *only* method that works reliably. This approach emphasizes learning new reasoning skills and techniques for achieving the winning attitude needed for success. Approaching weight-loss hurdles with reality-based optimism means keeping a calm head when things go wrong, and believing in your ability to pick yourself up and get right back on track. When you think rationally about setbacks you spare yourself from upsetting emotions. This frees your mind so that you can employ action-techniques to keep you from falling back into poor fitness habits and regaining weight.

> You must believe that you can pick yourself up and get back on track.

Your state of mind plays a determining role in your weight-loss success. When we lack confidence about reaching our goals, we are less likely to reach them. Feeling hopeless about being able to lose weight kills motivation. Losing weight is a journey that is wrought with ups and downs. Surviving the ups—the victories—is easy, but those who reach their weight goals are the people who weather the downs and spring back from setbacks. Pessimists interpret their setbacks in negative terms which undermines their ability to stop backsliding. Psychologists Bernard Weiner and Martin E.P. Seligman's work reveals that pessimists explain setbacks to themselves *as permanent, pervasive, and personal*—called the three P's of pessimism. Pessimists believe setbacks are *permanent*—"I'll never get the hang of this", *personal* —"It's just me—I have no willpower", and *pervasive*—"Since I've blown the diet, I may as well blow off the exercising too".

Optimists do the opposite. They see their setbacks as *temporary*, *specific* to the situation at hand, and *not* due to *personal* failing. This way of explaining events to oneself enables optimists to keep a cool head when dealing with setbacks so that they can get right back on track.

Check Your Attitude

NEGATIVE THINKING CAN MEAN SERIOUS TROUBLE in achieving our goals—weight-loss or otherwise! Go back to the weight-loss attitude quiz on page 12. Grab a pencil and circle all the items you rated as 3 or higher. Each item reflects one of the three pessimistic P's. Items 1, 4,

> Negative thinking gets in the way of achieving goals.

7 and 10 indicate that you view setbacks as pervasive—that is, you see a setback in one area as automatically leading to setbacks in other areas. The higher you rated these items the more you are likely to conclude that a setback in one area of your life is related to potential setbacks in other areas of your life. Items 2,5,8, and 11 reflect attitude towards permanent. If you rated these items as 3 or higher you tend to explain setbacks as being permanent.

If you rated items 3, 6, 9 and 12 as 3 or higher, you tend to interpret slip-ups as a sign of something being wrong with you. Losing weight is a challenge for all of us—not just for you. Three—P thinking is so insidious it often happens automatically. As you become more aware of your pessimistic thinking habits you will be more able to nip it in the bud and replace it with upbeat logic.

Weight-Loss Principles

THERE ARE THREE BASIC RULES to remember about losing weight. You must burn more calories than you take in, focus on sound nutrition, and cultivate a winning attitude.

Burn More Calories

CALORIES IN MINUS CALORIES OUT determines the amount of weight-loss. This principle is so basic that we often ignore it to chase hoaxes because we think it can't be this simple. It really is. If you are overweight, you are eating more calories than you are expending through exercise. It's as simple as that! Imagine you have a rubber oil tank in your basement, and the fuel truck comes to fill it up. If the oil truck continues pumping after the tank is full, the tank will expand as it accommodates the extra oil. Similarly, if you are putting too much "fuel" into your body through shoddy eating habits, which you aren't burning up through exercise, your thighs and belly will begin to expand just like that oil tank did. The key to losing weight is to cut down on the fuel deliveries—the amount of food you eat— and turn up the thermostat by exercising. Whenever you sweat from walking, running, or biking, you are burning up reserve fuel in your body.

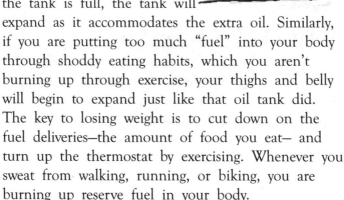

You Are What You Eat

GOOD NUTRITION IS ESSENTIAL. Your body needs clean nutrient-dense fuel to function like it should, especially when following a weight-loss diet. Clean fuel is food that is free of sugar, grease, chemicals, and dyes. Our wonderful bodies need vitamins, minerals, and the proper amount of healthy fats—like olive and flaxseed oil—in order to work efficiently. If we limit ourselves to one type of food, or lean heavily on sweets and coffee, we rob our cells of what they need to sustain healthy bones, muscles, and organs. In addition, our brains need nutrients to function. Washing down vitamin pills with coffee and doughnuts doesn't cut it. Vitamin supplements are meant to be additions—not substitutions—to a healthful daily food intake. Nothing can take the place of the nutrients found in nutritious foods, which act as the foundation for healthy, strong bodies.

See setbacks for what they really are.

Attitude is Everything

PERMANENT WEIGHT-LOSS is not only about eating and exercise. It is also about changing *your mind* to change your weight. This is what most weight-loss programs don't tell you. You know *what* to do and *how* to do it, but actually doing it depends on your attitude!

Attitude has a more powerful impact on weight-loss than any other single factor.

To normalize your weight once and for all, you must use optimistic thinking techniques. Psychological research is overwhelmingly clear on the benefits of using an optimistic thinking style when negative things happen. The most important benefit is resiliency—the ability to bounce back when the going gets tough in order to make it to the finish line. The key is to be rational about setbacks, and see them for what they really are—temporary, non-personal, isolated events. Optimistic thinking is a concrete skill that help you develop and maintain an attitude of *success*. I'm not talking about the "hooray for me" chants that deliver little and end up making us feel like fools. I am talking about specific ways of thinking about events that assist us in reaching our goals.

Thinking Style is Learned

YOU CAN LEARN TO THINK LIKE AN OPTIMIST, even if you are not an optimist by nature. You will benefit from incorporating optimistic thinking into all areas of your life. "Learned optimism", as Seligman calls the deliberate use of optimistic thinking, has helped millions of people achieve success in areas of health, education, and career. The kind of optimism you will learn here, is based on rational, positive thinking—not blind hope!

2

Optimism & Weight-Loss

PSYCHOLOGIST MARTIN E.P. SELIGMAN, renowned
for his work on Optimism Theory, demonstrated that pessimistic thinking promotes helplessness and depression, and produces inertia in
the face setbacks. Pessimism is also associated with
poor physical and psychological health.

When left unchallenged, pessimistic thinking can
take over your reasoning mechanisms. Before long,
you perceive everything that happens to you as
negative and hopeless; even when in reality, it may
be just the opposite. Fortunately, because helplessness is learned, it can be unlearned, and substituted
with a new way of thinking that generates hope
and determination. Optimistic thinking promotes
persistence, which is what helps you to re-mobilize
and get back on track after dieting and exercise
setbacks.

Thinking and Weight-Loss

OCCASIONAL SETBACKS are part and parcel of the
weight loss process—in fact, they are a natural part
of life. The probability of achieving your goals is

directly related to the way you account for your setbacks. To rebound effectively, you must remind yourself that setbacks are temporary, confined to the particular instance at hand, and not due to personal incompetence. In other words, you must learn to think like an optimist!

Knowing how to bounce back before setbacks get out of hand—such as a weight gain of 5 pounds, which turns into 20—will determine who gets fit and who stays fat. To do this, you must reason aggressively with yourself the moment you feel pummeled by your own negative thinking. Once you start explaining setbacks

Occasional setbacks are normal.

to yourself as temporary, confined to this one instance, and not a result of a personal defect, you will be happier, healthier, and more successful at anything you set out to do. Because losing weight is hard work and laden with challenges, optimism is the most important attribute to cultivate for anyone who is serious about getting fit.

Wishes into Reality

OVERSHOOTING WHAT YOU CAN REALISTICALLY ACHIEVE will leave you feeling drained if you can't meet your own expectations. Undershooting will also de-motivate you, because you won't see results fast enough. Be realistic about how much time and effort you think you can and will devote to weight-loss. Clearly, you know you will have to give it some elbow grease. How will you fit your fitness efforts in with the rest of your daily activities?

Reality-based optimism and self-efficacy will keep your motivational level steady by helping you to persevere until your goal is reached. Persistence is

95% of any battle. Remember the children's story of *The Little Engine That Could*? It is the story of a very small engine faced with the task of pulling a large broken-down train over a mountain. The Little Engine made several unsuccessful attempts at this seemingly impossible task, but refused to give up. Why did the Little Engine finally succeed? Because it *believed* it could. "I think I can, I think I can", the Little Engine told itself over and over, as it lugged the heavy train up the mountain. Now does this mean that all you have to do is chant "I will loose weight, I will loose weight" and you're there? Not so fast! Remember, there was no magic bullet. This is where the *reality* part comes in. The key is to say: "I know I can, I know I can—*and here's how I will do it!*"

Wishing alone won't help you lose weight, But knowing you are capable of doing the right things will! The "right things", include making small, steady adaptations in your eating and exercise habits, and keeping notes in your journal as to which strategies work and which don't.

No Frills Truths

OPTIMISM AND REALISM are not mutually exclusive; to the contrary, they should always go hand in hand. Reality-based optimism means keeping a rational, positive state of mind, especially when things go wrong. Reality is our friend. Optimism

Reality is a friend. doesn't mean lying to yourself or living in a state of denial where you ignore what you don't want to see. When you refuse to face reality, it is much harder to achieve your goals. There are ten realistic weight-loss strategies that we must accept from the start if we are to lose weight and keep it off.

Twelve Sure-Fire Strategies
for Shedding Pounds

1. Keep portion sizes to normal, single servings.
2. Drink 8-10 glasses of water each day.
3. Cut down on sugar, & refined carbohydrates.
4. Don't eat after dinner.
5. Exercise aerobically 30 minutes each day.
6. Lift weights 2-3 times a week.
7. Eat 7 servings of fruits & vegetables.
8. Don't snack; regulate your eating.
9. Cut out fried, fatty, and fast foods.
10. Reverse small weight gains right away.
11. Get up, get out, and move often.
12. Eat only when you are actually hungry.

These strategies seem deceptively mundane, yet they are based on the powerful truths of those who have been successful in losing weight and keeping it off. Diet books may skirt around these principles, but rarely come out and say, "No, you can't snack all day long and still lose weight! Nor can you eat endless amounts of fried dough pizza and doughnuts!" There is no getting around it—the bottom line is that you *must* eat fewer calories than you burn. Employing the twelve strategies will get you started on that path. Even if you don't want to count calories, you should be aware of the calorie count in basic foods—most people have no clue!

The twelve strategies are not always easy to follow, nor are they exciting. There is no magic to them. However they *do* work, and they work hand in hand with the mental restructuring that you are about to learn. Optimistic reasoning skills coupled with specific concrete actions will propel you right to the finish line. Stay clear of programs that tell you otherwise.

Change Your Mind, Change Your Weight

ABOUT 70 PERCENT OF US ARE OVERWEIGHT. Some of us suffer from obesity and its myriad of related illnesses. There are more overweight children now, than at any other time in history. As the decades pass, our weight is steadily climbing.

Being overweight is a life-threatening health risk and not just an aesthetic concern. Obesity is related to adult-onset diabetes, joint problems, certain cancers, coronary disease, stroke, emotional difficulties, job discrimination, loneliness, and more. In most cases, even a small weight loss can whisk you out of harm's way. But incredulously, we keep eating ourselves into self-destruction. We buy all the latest diet books, and reduced-calorie foods, yet we continue to get fatter and more frustrated than ever.

> Being overweight is a life-threatening health risk.

Some experts have boldly proclaimed that diets just don't work. At face value, this might seem reasonable. As a result of hearing this message, millions of overweight people felt they had psychological permission to give up, and as a result, stopped making any further attempts to lose weight. Giving up is certainly easier than facing the fact that losing weight takes hard work. The actual truth is—unsound diets don't work! When you accept your weight-loss challenge with determination and follow a

sound approach, you *will* end up with results to be
proud of. You may stumble again and again, but if
you give up, the road ends there, leaving you
helpless—and overweight.

Change Your Mind, Change Your Weight is a mind-
body approach designed specifically for those who
are ready to get down to
brass tacks and follow
a sound eating and
exercise plan. I won't
lie to you. To succeed
you must be ready to
"clean up your thinking". You must
make reality-based optimism a habitual part of your
thinking, especially as it pertains to your weight
loss. As your reasoning process changes, so will
your behaviors—and so will your weight.

As in learning any new skill, changing how you
think takes dedication and practice. You will zero
in on situations that have repeatedly caused you
difficulty. You will pinpoint the negative emotions
they elicit from you, then change them into positive
emotions that empower you. Finally, you will learn
to argue with your defeatest thinking. Just as you
would set the record straight with others who might
deride you, you will do the same with *yourself* the
next time you berate yourself about eating that
extra piece of chocolate cake. The realistic optimist
does not let slip-ups hold her down. Instead, slip-
ups will become challenges to overcome. The key
is to wipe out the irrational voice of failure and
replace it with a realistic voice of success. The
techniques you are about to learn will help you
change your weight—and your life.

3

Assess Your Readiness

D R. KELLY BROWNELL AND OTHER RESEARCHERS in the field of obesity believe that one of the most important predictors of weight loss success is one's psychological readiness to follow a weight-loss program. Dieting readiness is determined by several factors, including the tendency to let emotions, rather than physical hunger, determine eating patterns; motivation and commitment; and the presence of life events that might distract you from your weight-loss goals.

Determining ahead of time which factors might stand in the way of your losing weight gives you a chance to correct them so that you can focus your energy on getting fit. Once all systems are "go" you will move through the weight-loss process with much less difficulty.

Readiness

AS WITH ANY TASK, to succeed at losing weight you need to know what skills and behaviors are required. Then you can evaluate your strengths and weaknesses with respect to those skills. A *skill* is an acquired ability, and does not pertain only to physical capabilities. Restructuring one's mental activity from negative to positive is also an ability that can be developed with practice. Most people don't realize they can use their thoughts, feelings, and attitudes, to their advantage and that these positive attitudinal skills really hold the key to weight-loss success.

Confidence is a Booster

OUR THINKING STYLE ACTS AS A CATALYST to feelings of enthusiasm and confidence or feelings of fear and helplessness. The good news is that thinking style doesn't just happen—it is learned. How we feel and respond to situations, especially setbacks and disappointments, is learned. There is a clear connection between one's level of confidence and actual success in loosing weight.

Confidence is learned.

Fortunately, confidence is *learned.* Confident people are not born that way. They have learned through experience, to respond to difficulties and challenges in a positive and productive way, instead of doubting or berating themselves when they slip up. This reinforces their tenacity to handle future challenges with equal self-assuredness. The important point here is that mental attitude is a skill, and because skills are learned, we can learn new ways to think and feel, and thereby acquire the confidence we need to commit to our goals tenaciously.

Distractions Sidetrack Goals

STUDIES HAVE ALSO SHOWN that people are more likely to succeed at losing weight if they start their program when there are no other major distractions in their lives. Experiencing a major change or trauma—such as quitting smoking, changing jobs, or losing a loved one—require large amounts of energy and can often be stressful. Some people find it difficult to contemporaneously handle the stress of trying to lose weight. If this pertains to you, you might want to let some time pass in order to regroup your energy and mental resources, before starting a weight-loss program.

Emotional Eating Sabotages

BEING ABLE TO CONTROL EMOTIONAL EATING is essential for avoiding the unnecessary calories that pile up the pounds. Most of us fall prey to occasional emotion-driven eating, but if eating in reaction to your emotions is an overwhelming problem for you, you would be doing yourself a favor in seeking psychotherapy, which will help you to deal directly with the emotions that are causing you distress.

> Curtailing emotional eating is essential for permanent weight-loss.

How Ready Are You?

THE QUESTIONNAIRE THAT FOLLOWS is helps you evaluate your readiness to lose weight. Don't get hung up in "looking good" when answering the questions. This exercise is just for you. No one else will see it—unless you want to show it. While this is not a "scientific" assessment, the more honestly you respond, the greater insight you will gain on which areas you need to zero in on to achieve your goal. Your score may vary a little, each time you take it.

Are You an Emotional Eater?

Instructions: Recall your eating patterns for the last 6 months as you read the items. Using a scale from 1 to 5, with 1 being "rarely" and 5 being "usually," rate how often the following situations lead you to overeating.

Rarely   1   -   2   -   3   -   4   -   5   Usually

___1. When I am sad.
___2. When I am stressed.
___3. When I am happy.
___4. When I am angry.
___5. When I am bored.
___6. When I am frustrated.
___7. When I am lonely.
___8. When I see or smell food.
___9. When I am in social situations.
___10. When I see TV commercials.

Scoring:

40-50: Emotion-Driven Eater: You let emotions and other cues—rather than actual physical hunger—dictate your eating. Using food for reasons other than to fuel your body leads to a cycle of excess weight and negative emotions. You might conside talking to a psychotherapist to see what is really "eating" you. Once your emotional issues are resolved it will be easier for you to control overeating.

21-39: Middle-of-the-Road Emotional Eater: Whle you don't always eat in response to emotions, you do so often enough to sabotage your weight-loss efforts. Identify which emotions send you running to the refrigerator and write out a plan in your journal to substitute a healthy activity for eating when you catch wanting to eat when you are not hungry. This will bolster your ability to lose weight and keep it off.

10-20: Rational Hunger-Driven Eater: You rarely eat when you are not hungry. Still, be vigilant to not slip into emotional eating patterns when you are stressed and over-loaded. Make notes in your journal as to how you deal with specific emotions through-out the day, as a reminder to eat only when physically hungry.

Many of us eat in response to emotions and other internal and external associa-tions that have nothing to do with physical hunger. These associations include the sight and smell of food (external), or certain emotions that we feel (internal). An example is head-ing straight for the comfort foods when feeling depressed. Come to think of it, many of us head for those foods when we are feeling happy, too!

Eating in the absence of physical hunger serves as a temporary distraction for what is really ailing us. When this becomes a frequent occurrence, unless we deal with the root of the problem, the extra food will become problematic in itself and the pounds will pile on. To succeed at losing weight once and for all it is imperative to find non-edible ways to express anger, anxiety, depression, and happiness—and to respond without overeating to the sights, smells, and sounds of food. The objective is to move yourself from emotional eating to eating only when you are actually physically hungry.

Notice Bodily Signals

PAY ATTENTION TO BODILY SIGNALS. The first step in changing any behavior is being able to identify it, figure out what conditions lead up to it, and then come up with strategies for responding differently to these internal and external cues from this point on.

Compulsive eaters don't notice bodily signals of actual physical hunger.

Start by identifing the sensations you feel when you are physically hungry. Does your stomach growl? Does your head feel light? Sensations such as these, which indicate actual physical hunger, are the only signals that should lead you to eat. In contrast, identify which emotions or external temptations cause you to head for which foods? Do you gravitate toward salty, crunchy foods when you feel stressed? Do you grab a chocolate bar when feeling sad? Does a TV commercial for cola sent you running to the refrigerator for a can of soda? Make notes of all of these personal identifiers in your journal. The more you iron out possible obstacles ahead of time, the less difficulty you will face as you continue your journey towards a slimmer you.

How Distracting Is Your Life?

Instructions: Think of your life as it is now. Using a scale of 1 to 5, with 1 being "not likely" and 5 being "very likely," rate how likely it is that the situation in the item will occur in your life in the next six months.

Not Likely   1 - 2 - 3 - 4 - 5   Very Likely

__1. I will be getting married or divorced.
__2. I will quit smoking.
__3. I will change jobs.
__4. I will be moving.
__5. I will have a new member in my family.
__6. I will be separated from someone close.
__7. I will face a major health crisis.
__8. I will have gained or lost a pet.
__9. I will struggle with an emotional trauma.
__10. I will deal with a mental health issue.

Scoring:

40-50: High Life-Distraction Potential: Starting a weight-loss program may be unwise at this time because you are burdoned with considerable life-stress. Work on reducing the stressors in your life so that you can get on with your goals.

21-39: Moderate Life-Distraction Potential: Your current life situation has the potential to distract you from losing weight. With careful planning, you can reduce stress in your life. Get your journal and make a plan for staying focused on your weight-loss goals despite chaos in your life.

10-20: Low Life-Distraction Potential: Your life situation is stable and your weight-loss journey is not likely to be encumbered by distracting events. This is a good time to start and stick to a weight-loss program.

Major life stressors like quitting smoking, coping with a death in the family, or changing jobs, require most of your energy, leaving little left over for weight-loss commitment. Dealing with major changes and traumatic life events is always difficult and takes our attention away from other issues, like losing weight. Your ability to stay focused on your weight-loss efforts, despite life's stressors, will play a major role in your success. If you have a situation in your life right now that might distract you from staying committed to your weight-loss goals, this might not be the best time for you to start your program.

What is Your Behavior Change Confidence Level?

Instructions: Think ahead to a time when you are actively working to lose weight as you read the items. Using a scale from 1 to 5, with 1 being "unsuccessful" and 5 being "successful," rate how successful you expect to be at accomplishing the action   described in the item.

Unsuccessful 1 - 2 - 3 - 4 - 5 Successful

__1. I will eat only when I am actually hungry.
__2. I will reduce portion sizes.
__3. I will not eat sugary snacks.
__4. I will not eat fried foods.
__5. I will not eat fatty foods.
__6. I will not eat white-flour based products.
__7. I will drink 8-10 glasses of water a day.
__8. I will eat 7-10 servings of fruits & veggies daily.
__9. I will add physical activity to my daily activities.
__10. I will do 30 minutes of exercise daily.

Scoring:

10-20: You Are a Self-Doubter: Lack of confidence in your ability to do what it takes to lose weight stands between you and your goal. Developing a plan for accomplishing each item will help.

21-39: You Have Self-Doubter Potential: You may be doubting yourself to have an excuse in case you fail. To ensure against self-doubt and unnecessary difficulty, zero in on the items on which you scored a 3 or less and devise a plan to succeed in accomplishing these activities.

40-50: You Have High Confidence: You are not entrapped in senseless doubt. Instead, you believe in your ability to find solutions, which gives you a head start in reaching your weight-loss goals.

How Confident Are You in the Face of Setback?

Instructions: Think ahead to a time when you are actively working to lose weight. Read each item below and using a scale form 1 to 5, with 1 being "unsuccessful" and 5 being "successful" rate how successful you expect to be at accomplishing the action in the item.

Unsuccessful 1 - 2 - 3 - 4 - 5 Successful

__1. I will not blame myself if I go off my plan.
__2. I will be able to get right back on track.
__3. I will focus on weight-loss success stories.
__4. I will recall past successes to inspire me..
__5. I will reward myself for small improvement.
__6. I will actively encourage myself.
__7. I will set goals for small improvements.
__8. I will seek out people who encourage me.
__9. I will keep calm in the face of setback.
__10. I will plan ways to do better next time.

Scoring:
10-20: Setback Vulnerability: Setbacks unravel you and make you give up too easily. Resist becoming a victim of self-doubt by taking immediate action. Instead focus on the ways you successfully negotiate challenges you build self-confidence.

21-39: Setback Master Potential: Setbacks can potentially determine your fate. You have a moderate tendency to buckle in the face of setbacks, which unchecked, could deplete your resources of valuable energy you could be using toward reaching your goals. Examine items in which you could stand some improvement and work on them to help change your reaction to setback.

40-50: Setback Master: You turn obstacles into challenges to overcome and refuse to let everyday slip-ups keep you down. Your ability to get right back into the game will help you find you way to the finish line.

Do you keep telling yourself "I think I can't"? If so, now is the time to boost your self-confidence. One way to do this is by recalling your past successes, observing others succeed at the same task, surrounding yourself with people who encourage you, and staying calm about doing what is required.

Recall Past Success

WHEN YOU HAVE SUCCEEDED AT SOMETHING in the past, you will be more confident about succeeding at a similar task in the future. This point drives home the rationale for starting out small. Start with small actions you can master, like walking for 10 minutes a day, or drinking one extra glass of water a day. These small successes will make you

feel confident that you can do more of the same—
and perhaps a little bit more after that. Don't
think of weight-loss as a fixed number somewhere
out on the horizon. Instead, think of your goal-
weight as an accumulation of small individual
health-promoting behaviors that you do one at a
time, every day. Thus, instead of the 50 pounds
you will lose some day, focus on the 10-minute
walk or the extra glass of water that you can imple-
ment today. Soon you will build up a repertoire of
successful "past" performances that will produce
more of the same in the future.

Look for Success Models

WHEN WE WATCH OTHERS SUCCEED at something we
are striving for, we feel more confident about the
likelihood of our own success. We all know someone who has succeeded in losing weight. If you
don't, there are plenty of autobiographical accounts
at your local bookstore.
Study these cases carefully.
Read about how they
achieved their weight goals.

> The mind constantly thinks "can do" or "can't do."

You will identify more personally with someone's
success if his or her situation is similar to yours.
Most people love to share their "secrets."

Stay Calm and Ready

EMOTIONAL STATE INFLUENCES CONFIDENCE. Sometimes
being slightly anxious about the task ahead is
helpful. It keeps us alert and ready. However, too
much worry or anxiety is counterproductive, and
causes us to fumble when attempting to reach our
goals. The weight-loss process can be a stressful
pursuit to begin with, not to mention the stress
associated with work, family, and everyday hassles.

We all need to learn how to de-stress. There are many effective stress management classes we can avail ourselves of. We can also learn about meditation, visualization, and relaxation breathing techniques by visiting your local bookstore. Remaining calm during difficulty increases our chances of overcoming that difficulty.

How Prepared Are You to Loss Weight?

Instructions: Think ahead to a time when you are beginning your weight-loss program. Read each item and, using a scale from 1 to 5, with 1 being "not willing" and 5 being "very willing" rate how willng you will be to carry out the action in the item.

Not willing   1 - 2 - 3 - 4 - 5   Very willing

__1. I will remove snack foods from the house.
__2. I will tell family and friends of my plans.
__3. I will evaluate several programs first.
__4. I will select a program that fits my lifestyle.
__5. I will select a program that yields slow loss.
__6. I will discuss my program with my doctor.
__7. I will keep a written log of my progress.
__8. I will do 30 minutes of exercise a day.
__9. I will resolve distracting life situations.
__10. I will seek help for issues that interfere.

Scoring:

10-20: You Are in Denial: You aren't convinced that you can achieve your weight-loss goal. Weight-loss takes careful preparation. Your efforts will pay off when you make a commitment to doing what it takes to lose weight.

21-39: You are a Fledging Realist: You seem willing to do pre-planning. To give yourself the maximum chance for success, you must built each action described in the tiems into your planning.

40-50: You are a Smart Planner. You expect to do pre-planning and understand the time you spend preparing in advance will make the journey to weight-loss that much easier.

Making well thought-out preparations before starting a weight-loss program gives you a powerful edge toward success. Be prepared to forego fad diets that promise unrealistically high weight-loss in a short time, which will leave you feeling more frustrated when the pounds find their way back onto your hips and thighs. Instead, expect to lose weight slowly—1.5 to 2 pounds a week, which is sensible and realistic. Explore the free resources at your library and on the Internet to find a sensible diet and exercise plan.

> Anticipating and planning for difficulties makes it easier to lose weight.

After you have carefully chosen an eating and exercise plan that works with your lifestyle, discuss it with your physician to make sure it fits with your general health care planning. Remember that the thought and effort you put into your project before beginning your program will save you from needless mistakes down the line. Don't cringe at the thought of a little extra work. Instead embrace the work you put into weight-loss preparation—it is testimony to your commitment to the most important person on earth—you!

4

Keep A Journal

MAKE SURE THAT YOUR EXPECTATIONS are realistic or you will get discouraged and give up before long. If you think you *should* be able to lose large amounts of weight each week, or that you will never have moments in which you want to eat more than you *should*—think again! Instead, prepare yourself—realistically—for what lies ahead, then half the battle is won. One way to keep yourself "real" is to keep a daily log.

What to Do

Buy a blank book or notebook to use for evaluating your weight-loss readiness, developing your goals and keeping track of your progress. This will help you to

> Keeping a journal helps to identify the relaitonship between your actions and your weight-loss.

better grasp the relationship between your actions and your weight-loss patterns. The notebook will be used to keep a diary or daily log of your actions, thoughts, feelings, ideas, and progress related your weight-loss goals. Consistently writing in your journal will bring clarity to your thoughts and actions, and reveal what needs to be done to reach your goals. Sometimes we get so bombarded with non-essential thoughts and information, that we don't remember where we are or where we're going. Your journal will tell you where you've been and where you are going, every step of the way.

Some people think they eat too little to be overweight and mistakenly believe their weight gain is due to a metabolic disorder. When they document everything they eat in their journal along with all of their exercise activities, they discover they have been sabotaging themselves.

Self-Sabotage

SELF-SABOTAGING BEHAVIORS include anything you do that undermines achieving your goals. For instance, calories are calories, and anything you put into your mouth that is not on your eating plan, still counts as extra food and calories! Thus, you sabotage yourself when you "take just a taste" while cooking, or when you "just finish the few crumbs" at the bottom of the cookie jar. Other insidious calories come from licking the spoon after frosting the cake, tasting supermarket display samples, eating a couple of cookies while doing your work at the computer, and taking a second portion of food at the supper table. Many of these behaviors come so automatically to us that we are barely conscious of them—and then we wonder why the scale refuses to go down! In keeping a journal, you will be

> You sabotage yourself when you "have just a taste."

documenting all of these subtle deviations from your eating plan, so you will have no doubt as to exactly what is going on and what you need to do. No one need ever read the journal but you, so be as honest as you can. The information you glean from it will serve you well.

Jog Your Memory

PEOPLE WHO ARE OVERWEIGHT typically underestimate what they eat. Most of us believe we eat far less than we do, and forget about the small extras that build up calories.

> Overweight people tend to underestimate how much they have eaten.

The same thing happens with exercise. You may think you got enough exercise today, when all you really did was walk up the flight of stairs from the basement. Taking control of your life starts with *awareness* of the activity as you engage in it. That awareness comes from writing down your thoughts and actions throughout the day. Otherwise we go through much of our day in a state of semi-awareness. If you don't believe how much of everyday life sails by unnoticed, try this exercise:

A Penny for Your Thoughts

On a blank sheet of paper draw a detailed sketch of a penny—just the head side. Include everything you can remember. Who is the figurehead on your penny? In which direction is the head facing? Is there anything written over the head? If so, what? Is there any writing or images to the left and/or right? If so, what are those words or images? After you have done this, take out a real penny and check your accuracy.

If you are like most people who do this exercise, you will have made at least a few errors! Don't feel bad; it is simply a matter of what we pay attention to. When we don't give something our full attention, it rarely stays in our memory bank. As you can tell from this penny exercise, you can see something every day and not notice the details.

Journaling helps you notice the details. Journaling helps you notice the details. You will begin to notice—and take control of—things like consuming extra calories, emotional eating, and the physical exercise you are *really* getting on a daily basis. Journaling forces us pay attention, so we won't be stumped as to why we haven't lost weight, despite our efforts. Better yet, we will clearly be able to figure out what we should do next, in order to get results.

Journal Elements

CONSIDER YOUR JOURNAL as a personalized book to be referred to again and again whenever you need to reverse small or large weight gains. Here are a few elements to include in your daily journal:

Time Line

RECORD EACH HOUR OF THE DAY along the left hand margin, starting with the time you get up, and ending with the time you go to bed. You may divide your timeline into half hour segments as well—for example 8am, 8:30am, and so on. Record the precise times that you eat, exercise, snack, and experience negative feelings. Record your weight-loss related actions (eating and exercise) and feelings, next to the appropriate half-hour interval. This will give you a better defense against emerging or existing difficulties in these areas.

Situation

MAKE SURE TO RECORD SITUATIONS in which you overeat. Who were you with? What were you doing? Where were you physically situated (kitchen table, restaurant, in front of the TV, etc.)? Full awareness of the situation in which you typically overeat is the first step towards breaking the association between situation and automatic eating.

Food consumption

WRITE DOWN EVERY MORSEL that you consume. Include the cookie crumbs you polished off before throwing the bag away, the handful of peanuts you swiped from your son's after school snack, the spoonful of pudding you tasted just to make sure it came out right. You will not be showing this diary to anyone, so be honest with yourself.

Planned Exercise Sessions

RECORD THE TIME OF DAY YOU EXERCISED, the type of exercise you did, and the amount of time it took you to complete it. Then rate each exercise daily on a scale from one to five, five being "thoroughly enjoyed it", one being "hated it". In general, you will stick with a routine that you enjoy. If you are doing exercise that is too hard or too easy for you, or based on an activity that you never liked to begin with, it is a matter of time before you abandon ship!

Lifestyle Activity

REMEMBER CALORIES IN MUST BE LESS than calories out if your goal is to lose weight. List all the activities you do throughout the day that keep your body in motion. Include everything from taking that extra flight of stairs, to that half-hour of weeding the garden. Write down additional ideas about how to start burning more calories by making some minor changes in your daily routine.

Monitor Emotions

MANY THINGS THAT HAPPEN in the course of a day elicit emotional reactions. Eating and exercising often produce certain feelings. We also respond to interactions with people at work, and to phone conversations with salespeople who won't take "no" for an answer, for example. A song on the radio can bring up memories from the past. Noticing your emotional reactions is an important step in building the positive thinking style we are aiming for. Document any notable emotions, along with the time, place, and the situation under which you experienced these emotions. Note why you were upset, anxious, depressed, or experienced other strong feelings.

Setting Up the Journal

SET UP YOUR JOURNAL ANYWAY YOU LIKE. Here are some general tips. Use a spiral notebook, a bound blank page book, or a 3 ring binder. Don't use individual sheets of paper, because the continuity will get lost if you lose some pages. Here is a sample journal layout. Notice that it includes all of the key information, such as the time and the situation under which you ate, exercised, and experienced emotion. You can write down additional thoughts in the *reflections* section at the end of each page.

Sample Journal Page

Time	Situation	Food	Exercise	Emotion
7:30	Sister visited	3 Cookies & coffee		Guilt
8:15			30-min walk	Joy
9:20	Sitting at table	Apple		Satisfied

Reflections: *I feel better when I stick to my plan. The pleasure of eating the cookies wasn't worth the guilt.*

Be as detailed as you would like, but don't let keeping a journal become drudgery. Keep notations short and simple. Keep the journal handy, so that you can use it often. A pocket size notebook is more portable. You can keep it in your purse or glove compartment, and write down your thoughts and activities more frequently throughout the day.

Fine-Tuning

ANALYZING THE NOTATIONS IN YOUR JOURNAL will help you to get to know yourself better. It will also will help you to avoid massive setbacks by continually refining your goals and behaviors. Before you go to bed, set aside five to ten minutes to reflect upon the day's journal entry. Note where you had difficulty, and which weight-loss techniques came easy for you. You might use a yellow marker to highlight what went according to your plan, and a different color marker to bring your attention to problem areas. Figure out why you experienced difficulty. Look for patterns. Is there a certain time of day when you automatically snack without think-ing? Is there a particular situation—like having an unexpected visitor—that causes you to eat more than you wanted to? Perhaps your weight goal was unre-alistic, and needs to be modified. Maybe your eating and exercise plan needs to be refined. Write all of this down in the *reflections* section at the end of each day in your notebook. Make notes on how you can make little strides forward for the next day. Gradually, before you know it, you will have made one giant leap towards achieving your goal.

Keeping a log might seem like drudgery in the beginning but after a week or so you will become proficient at zeroing in on the important informa-tion to record. Keep sentences brief and to the point and always review your notes with an eye towards taking the next step forward.   Consider what you can do better tomorrow. Write down the small changes you can make in order to avoid the pitfalls your experienced today. Used in this way, journaling helps you make sense of your past weight-loss behaviors in order to make your future actions more precise and powerful.   The few min-utes you invest each day in writing will yield ben-efits well worth the time and effort that it takes.

5

Make A
Realistic Plan

CLEAR AND ORGANIZED PLAN for weight-loss is essential, because what goes on in your head influences what you do. You want what goes on in your head to have clarity, so you will know exactly what to do at all times. Solid planning and preparation lead to clear, calm thinking–an essential component for weight-loss success! The key is to marry mind and behavior and get them working seamlessly together.

Start with a simple, sensible eating and exercise program. There are many sensible programs that work, which are easy enough to follow. Regardless of which approach you choose, however, there are some basic guidelines that are useful in deciding how to eat and exercise for weight loss.

Select a Plan

IN SELECTING AN EATING PLAN you can live with, first consider a plan that is low in fat *and* sugar. Often low-fat foods are loaded with sugar and insidious calories that add up. Also, make sure your diet does not forbid fats *entirely*, because the body needs small amounts of healthy oils–such as olive or flaxseed oil–to function properly.

If you are a vegetarian, your eating plan will focus on plant-based foods, such as vegetables and fruits; legumes; whole grains; and low fat dairy, soy or wheat products for extra protein. If you are not _____ a vegetarian, you will still want to Solid planning is look for healthy protein sources your foundation. such as fish, poultry, and occasion- _____ ally some lean red meat. Check with your doctor about taking a multivitamin, and possibly a calcium supplement, if appropriate. Make sure the eating plan you choose makes it easy for you to eat in restaurants without gaining weight, and is not so low in calories that you feel hungry all day.

Check with Your Physician

LOSING WEIGHT STRAINS YOUR BODY. Make sure to rule out conditions that might put your health at risk when you lose weight. Show your doctor the weight-loss and exercise program you decided to follow. She might be able to advise you as to how to better adapt it to your medical needs. If you have been for a physical checkup within the past 6 months, a simple phone call to your doctor may suffice.

Lifestyle Exercise

THERE IS AN IMPORTANT DISTINCTION between pro-grammed exercise and lifestyle activity. Programmed exercise refers to your daily planned aerobic or weight lifting sessions. Realize however, that no matter how conscientious you are about sticking to your programmed exercise, you will sabotage your weight-loss efforts if you remain sedentary for the rest of the day!

Get up from the computer or from in front of the TV and take frequent, active breaks. March in place, do a few jumping jacks, walk downstairs to take the laundry out of the dryer—every little bit helps! Lifestyle activity means movement—anywhere you can fit it in *throughout the day*. For example, instead of taking three or four bags of groceries from the car to the house to save yourself steps, always try to find ways to *increase* your steps! Take one bag of groceries from the car to the house at a time, or park in a space that is farther, rather than closer to your destination. If the mailbox is only a few blocks away, get those sneakers out and let your feet do the walking. There are countless ways to squeeze extra bits and pieces of lifestyle activity into your day. Be creative! Think *healthy* and your weight will normalize.

> Eating healthfully and exercising consistently are the most direct means you have of influencing your own health. And they are *both* under your control!

Plan for Tomorrow

REVIEW THE DIFFICULTIES YOU PINPOINTED and modify your plan to take those into account. Find solutions to those difficulties. Think through what you will eat, and what exercises you plan to do tomorrow. For example if you find you keep talking yourself out of the early morning jogs you had planned for, write out some possible thoughts as to why you resist them. Perhaps you are a person who never liked to get up early to begin with. Would a change to a later time correct the problem? Perhaps you never really liked jogging, or you have a bad knee that makes it painful to keep this commitment. Think of an alternate form of exercise you can switch to that would take these factors into account.   Preparation, such as writing out your plans ahead of time in your journal, puts the following day under your control. Regaining control of your life empowers you to succeed, and immunizes you against helplessness and depression.

Make a Commitment

MOST OF US WOULD NEVER BREAK a promise to a family member or to a close friend. When we give our word, we make good on it, and that's all there is to it. We like the feeling of being known as someone people can count on. Yet, when you stop to consider the relationship you've had with your body over the years, including the many times you started to get in shape then didn't follow through, can you honestly say that you have been there for yourself? It is imperative that you think of yourself as your closest friend and family member. The promises you make to yourself should be held sacred, and kept above all else. Believe in your ability to work hard for yourself. Then do it!

Believe in yourself!

Deciding on an exercise plan is easy if you remember to include the three fundamental components of fitness: aerobic activity, weight-lifting, and stretching. Your program should start out slow and build up to 30-45 minutes of aerobic activity on most days of the week. This could include brisk walking, running, swimming, cycling, skating, aerobic dance, or even jumping rope. For your bones and muscles you will have to lift at least some light weights a couple of times a week. This doesn't mean you have to buy an expensive gym membership. A couple of 5 to 10 pound dumbbells that you can store under the bed can be just as effective, and will cost a whole lot less.

In addition to stretching after your planned exercise activities, you may want to check out a Yoga class for its stretching benefits as well as for its relaxation effect, which is something we all could use when trying to lose weight.

Give Motivation a Boost

TO SUCCEED IN ANYTHING, you must consistently do what it takes to get there, even when you don't feel like it. We get up and go to work at a certain time—even on mornings we would rather sleep in. We grit our teeth and walk the dog—even in sub-zero degree weather. We don't need motivational techniques to do certain things; we simply do them because we have an obligation to fulfill. Start thinking of your health as the most important obligation of all. There will be days when you just have to clench your teeth and do what you have to do anyway, because you have an obligation to yourself to take care of your body.

Pressing for too much weight in too short of a time is a set up to fail.

Many factors determine motivational strength. These factors include how capable we think we are at succeeding; how reachable our goal is; what we expect to get out of reaching that goal; and how strong our need to achieve the goal is. Always set small gradual weight-loss goals that are within your capability to achieve. Be reasonable as to what to expect from your efforts (e.g., slow and steady weight loss and greater fitness). Remember that if you want it bad enough, nothing can stop you from finding your way to success.

Encouragement

WE FEEL STRONGER and more confident about sticking to your plan when others encourage us and believe in our ability to succeed. Seek the company of people who make you feel good. Surround yourself with positive people who care about you, whether you are losing weight or not. Certain family members may fit the bill, as may one or two of your closest friends. When a person whom we trust roots for us, we tend to internalize their encouragement. Their belief in us makes us believe in ourselves.

When encouragement is not forthcoming, ask for it. "How am I doing?" is a question you should never be ashamed to ask. Feedback is one of the most important reasons we socialize—we need the opinions and ideas of people whom we trust!

Stay Calm and Ready

EMOTIONAL STATE CAN INFLUENCE CONFIDENCE. Sometimes being slightly anxious about a task is helpful. It keeps us alert and ready. But too much worry or anxiety is counterproductive, and causes us to fumble when attempting to reach our goals. The weight-loss process is a stressful pursuit to begin with. We all need to learn how to de-stress. There are many effective stress management classes available. Learn about meditation, visualization, and relaxation breathing techniques by visiting your local bookstore. Remaining calm during difficulty increases our chances of overcoming that difficulty.

Getting feedback is one of the reasons we socialize.

Research shows that weight-loss confidence is associated with greater success in actually losing weight and sticking with your sound diet and exercise plans.

6

PERSONALIZE YOUR GOALS

CUSTOMIZING YOUR EXERCISE and eating program is important to losing and keeping weight off. The more your program is individually tailored, the more tenacious you will be about sticking with it. Weight-loss goals should always be reasonable, and centered around immediate, achievable behaviors that promote physical fitness. For example, "I will cut out all desserts", is a long-term goal. "I will cut out dessert at supper tonight", is an immediate, specific step that is easily achievable. This kind of goal will keep you motivated to do a little bit more the next time.

Goal-setting expert Dr. Beverly Potter warns about setting goals that are either too stringent, or not in line with who we really are. When your goal is poorly fitted to what you are capable of doing—or willing to do—you are likely to fail. Sure, you may be able to whip yourself into shape for a little while, but you'll probably give up along the way, or find yourself so exhausted at the finish line, that you won't enjoy the fruits of your efforts.

> Poorly fitting goals set you up to fail.

Keep your weight-loss goals small and achievable. The success you experience in reaching them will keep your motivation strong for reaching the end-goal—a physically-fit, healthy new you!. It is important to make peace with your body every step of the way. A lack of self-acceptance can cause us to set unrealistic goals that set us up to fail. For instance, when we disdain how we look, we are more prone to follow an overly restrictive diet, or exercise obsessively. A poor body image can also lead to eating-disordered behavior.

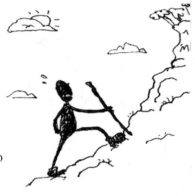

Body Image

POOR BODY IMAGE is becoming the norm. When we dislike how we look, we are more prone to experience low self-esteem, anxiety, depression, and eating disorders. Mass media's relentless attempts to convince us that we should be unrealistically thin, exacerbates the problem, as does constantly comparing ourselves to others who are better looking, slimmer, more muscular—more everything— than we are. Having been teased about our weight or appearance in our youth, also influences the way we feel about ourselves in adulthood. Increasingly more men and children are unhappy about their appearance, too. Although traditionally more women than men dislike their body, the gender gap is narrowing steadily.

Negative attitudes, perceptual distortions, and self-defeating behaviors directed toward our appearance, drive us to select "get thin quick" schemes. Marcia is a case in point. The first thing she does in the morning is look at herself in a full-length mirror and think, "Just look at these thunder thighs! I need to loose at least 40 pounds!" In reality Marcia is about 20 pounds overweight, but because she dislikes her thighs, she interprets the situation as much worse than it really is. She has a distorted perception about how overweight she is, which is often part of the body image disturbance syndrome, as is dragging out the "fat" clothes. Because of her tendency to exaggerate the problem, she put herself on a fad liquid diet, which inevitably she was not able to stick with.

Attitude, perception, and behavior are so intertwined that we hardly notice the interplay. Negative thoughts and self-deprecatory judgments influence the quality of your daily life. When you start your day by telling yourself how unattractive or unworthy you are, there is actually a change of brain chemistry that encourages negative thoughts to get recycled in your head all throughout the day. In contrast, putting on a smile and telling yourself good things changes brain chemistry, too—as well as your quality of life.

> Negative thoughts and self-deprecatory judgments spoil quality of life.

Smiling and seeing the positive aspects of yourself—even when you don't feel like it—will actually make you feel happier and more positive. If you head straight to your mirror and smile right now, you will notice almost an immediate change in the way you feel. If you're like most of us, you will feel just a little more cheerful after smiling for several seconds. Smiling bolsters your mood and increases your confidence. Since research confirms that facial expressions actually do create changes in the brain, perhaps it might just make tackling those saddlebags, easier too!

Body image disturbance is responsible for our insatiable appetite for plastic surgery, cosmetic potions, abdominal gizmos and miracle-diets-in-a-capsule. We are suckers for anything that will help us feel better about ourselves. What ultimately makes us feel better, though, doesn't come from anything outside of ourselves—like new gimmicks, or perfect mirror images. Feeling good about ourselves requires genuine self-respect and acceptance. Treat your body right—whatever its size. If you think "healthy", instead of "skinny," your goals will fall into line with what is right for you.

Obesity researchers use the term "reasonable weight", to refer to the weight that is realistically attainable for you, and which optimizes your chances of staying healthy and living longer. People

> Focus more on how you feel and less on how you look.

who feel healthy are not as likely to obsess about an extra inch here or there. If you focus more on how you feel and less on how you look, you will lose weight with much less trauma.

Reasonable Weight

REMEMBER, THE GOAL IS TO GET FIT and healthy, not to make yourself underweight or sickly. If your goal weight is too low, you will not be able to stick to that weight, even if you are able to achieve it. There are several ways to determine what is a reasonable weight for you.

Body mass index (BMI) is a calculation based on your weight in kilograms divided by your height in meters squared. This formula is highly correlated with body fat. There are free charts and guidelines on the Internet, which will give you an idea what your BMI should be.

Insurance company height and weight tables   are based on longevity calculations. They will frequently give you a range, which can serve as a rough guideline as to a reasonable weight for you.

Genetics are a reality. If your parents and other close relatives are overweight or obese, you might have to struggle more with weight than your genetically thin friends will. That doesn't mean there's no hope. On the contrary, those relatives may simply have had poor eating habits. Whatever the case, healthy habits and healthy thoughts will make a big difference in determining your weight and level of physical fitness. You just can't expect to look like a waif model if your genetic legacy is the opposite. The price you would have to pay to get there and stay there would make your life miserable.

Intuition is a reliable guide. You intuitively know what weight feels good to you. Again, think "healthy" and "fit". The weight at which you feel energetic, physically strong, and capable of maintaining without struggling, is probably your natural, reasonable weight.

Expectations can undermine your resolve. Focus on healthy *thoughts*, and individual *behaviors* that add up to physical fitness. The numbers on the scale will drop in their own time. In general, if you are losing more than 1-2 pounds a week, you are only loosing water, and water weight always comes back. Go slow, and monitor your sense of well-being.   Unrealistic weight-loss goals will only frustrate you.

The scale fluctuates with your body fluids, and when you see the scale go up despite having done everything you could to follow your plan, you will want to head for the hills screaming. Don't do it!

Think only of the individual activities you can do to stay on course, regardless of what the scale says. Will you walk for thirty minutes today? If that is not realistic, how about starting with ten minutes, then increasing to 20 minutes next week? This can constitute one of your small attainable goals, which, when put together with other small attainable goals, spell weight loss. Your behavior is something you can control—and so are your thoughts. The number on the scale, however, is not always under your control.

Set Small Goals

BREAKING LARGE GOALS INTO SMALLER, DOABLE SUBGOALS is a technique called "shaping". For example, when a goal seems too far away or intangible—for example, having thin thighs—we lose motivation to stick with it. We can derive a sense of self-efficacy, when we take that far-away goal and chop it up into little bits or sub-goals that are easily accomplished—doing

Break large goals into smaller, doable subgoals.

five minutes of squats each day may be one of the smaller sub-goals required for attaining the more distal goal of thinner thighs.

Success has a way of snowballing—and so does failure. Past accomplishments predict future accomplishments. For the person who generally doesn't like sweets and eats them only occasionally, cutting out sweets altogether might be a small, immediate, and doable goal. On the other hand, if you are used to eating sweets several times a day, it will not be so easy to do away with them all at once. Sugar has an addictive quality. Many of us can't have just one cookie, and need to weed sugar out of our diets more gradually. You might, for example, allow yourself dessert once a day for a while, so that your goal is simply to cut sweets out at lunchtime. Then, when you have accomplished that, you can cut out sugar at suppertime, too. Eventually, you can go further to eliminate desserts altogether.

Dealing with Setbacks

THERE ARE NO REAL FAILURES IN LIFE—only opportunities to learn. Fortunately humans have the ability to self-reflect. If you are having trouble reaching your goals, you must first ask yourself if they were attainable to begin with. Were your standards too stringent? Was the finish line so far away that you couldn't taste the fruits of your efforts? If so, then readjust and re-parse your goals into small, bite size pieces which are more appropriate for you.

Focusing on specific, doable actions as opposed to an intangible long-range target—like "loosing 50 pounds"—gives a sense of immediate control, which is fundamental to developing a winning attitude. Relax, and remember that the tortoise wins the race. Even small weight losses

Failures are opportunities to learn.

of as little as 10 to 15 percent of your starting weight helps reduce obesity-related maladies, such as hypertension, diabetes, depression, and low self-esteem.

7

Argue With Negativity

MYRA WENT TO A BUFFET-STYLE WEDDING party with a sumptuous spread, catered to perfection, complete with hot and cold salads, fried chicken, and roast beef with gravy—an "all-you-can-eat" paradise. Myra said to herself, "Oh no, this buffet is too much. Look at all that great food! Oh, what the heck, I don't do this everyday. I can always start again tomorrow, right? I'm digging in." Hesitating, Myra replied to herself, "Damn it, you blew it again! How long have you been on this diet anyway, all of 3 minutes? Face it, you were just meant to be heavy." "Who cares," Myra argued back, " I'm going to eat this whole damn table. I'll never lose weight anyway. Maybe there *is* something wrong with me.

Myra's thought process is problematic. We all have similar internal dialogues when faced with temptation. We are human, after all, and humans occasionally give in to temptation and fall off the wagon. This is to be expected. The key is to have a strategy to turn our setbacks into victories. Myra's giving into temptation to "pig out" when trying to stick to a weight loss plan is easy to relate to. We've all had this struggle. Conquering out of control eating is one of the most important things you can do to control your weight.

Positive Rebuttles

WHEN FACED WITH A SITUATION like Myra's we can decide to avoid similar situations altogether in the future, and never go to another buffet again; stuff ourselves for the moment and think about starting anew tomorrow; or just give up, because the temptation of food is stronger than we are. There is one strategy that will work better than any of those. Argue with yourself to arrive at a reasonable solution. Arguing with negative thoughts works!

Positive rebuttals to negative self-talk helps you stay on track without getting discouraged. You can turn setbacks into successes by refusing to obey those critical voices inside your head. Fight the voices that tell you that you messed up because there is something wrong with you (*personal*); that you messed up this time, therefore you are bound to mess up again (*permanent*); or that your slip-up is sure to spread to other areas of your life (*pervasive*).

Keep yourself from slumping into defeat, by figuring out realistic explanations as to *why* you slipped up. Put your reasoning in non-personal, non-permanent, and non-pervasive terms. Then come up with a concrete plan to put into action *next* time. Always put a dose of reality into your reasoning. You might have slipped up because of the situation, the food, or a temporary mood you were in—but never because of an inherent defect in you. Likewise, remember that falling off the wagon does not mean you are forever doomed to do the same.

Whenever you slip up, think of it as a non-permanent situation, pertaining to this one time only. Finally, don't generalize the slip up to other areas in your life. If you eat more than you should have, that doesn't mean you will also mess up at work. How logical is that? Yet many of us reason this way unconsciously.

Finish the Fight

DON'T LET THE THOUGHTS INSIDE YOUR HEAD linger on a sour note of helplessness that will haunt you throughout your day. Negativity is a psychological poison that pervades your subconscious and makes you feel helpless and depressed. Setbacks are normal and to be expected. Engage realistic optimism to put them into perspective, by taking control of your thoughts, your emotions, and your behavior. *Argue* with negative thoughts.

Myra's internal dialogue changed completely when she argued with her negative voices. "For heaven's sake. In *reality* all I did was eat some extra food at a single buffet. The food looked scrumptious and the people all around me were eating it with gusto. The problem is not *me*, it was the situation—which would have been tough for anyone to resist (non-personal). Next time, I will plan out what to eat ahead of time (finds a solution). I will make sure I cut out some of my calories during the day, so I can enjoy a little more food at the buffet. This way temptation won't catch me off guard. I don't have to lose

Talking back to negative thinking helps to get you back on track.

control when faced with food. Blowing it once doesn't mean I'll blow it every time (non-permanent). It is kind of silly to think that overeating at a buffet means everything in my life is jinxed (non-pervasive). Ok, now my head is on straight. I really feel better. That slip-up was not the end of the world."

Myra's original dialogue created a state of mind that turned a small mistake into a full-blown *permanent* failure, but when she argued back she felt energized and empowered. She successfully stopped herself from thinking irrationally and pessimistically about overeating at the buffet. Optimists see setbacks as non-personal, temporary, and specific to the situation at hand. That is why optimistic thinking helps us bounce back from defeat and avoid falling victim to feelings of longer-term helplessness.

> Think optimistically to bounce back from defeat.

8

ABC's of Weight-Loss

O CHANGE YOUR BEHAVIOR, the rule of thumb is "Use your ABC's". When examining the dynamics of upsetting situations, the ABC technique is used in settings from schools to prisons as well as weight-loss programs.

Weight-Loss ABC's

A = **Antecedent** or event that occurs, which usually unpleasant, stressful, or frightening.

B = **Belief** or thought about A, which is often erroneous or irrational

C = **Consequences** are the emotions or actions triggered by B.

The upsetting event (A) that occurred in Myra's overeating episode was giving in to temptation at the buffet. Because of this she told herself (B) that she "blew it," that there was something wrong with her, and that nothing she could do would amount to anything good. The emotional consequence (C) was a feeling of helpless, depression, and defeat.

Rational Thinking

WE ALL FALL PREY to self-defeating thinking patterns at one time or another. For many of us, it is an automatic process—we are not even conscious of it happening! Fortunately, this trend can be reversed—no matter how deeply pessimism has been ingrained in us—when we learn to think rationally and

> You can change habitual self-defeating thinking.

positively. Habitual self-defeating thinking patterns *can* be changed. It is not hard to make positive modifications in your thinking. Be courageous enough to argue with your catastrophic thinking!

In truth there are very few setbacks in life from which we can't recover. To combat self-defeating thoughts, add D & E to your ABC's. Dr. Albert Ellis who developed Rational Emotive Behavior Therapy uses the ABCDE's as a simple method to transform self-defeating thinking into rational thinking.

Dispute & Energize

D= Disputation of the irrational or pessimistic belief (B)

E= Energization, noticing and recording how much better you as a result of changing the negative belief

Dispute

DISPUTE (D) ALL BELIEFS that weaken your motivation to succeed by seeking evidence to the contrary, and looking for alternative solutions that empower you. For example, if your cousin convinces you to eat a large piece of cake, you might give in to avoid being rude, but then go home and berate yourself for lacking willpower. Instead, dispute the belief that you have no willpower, then think of a solution to handle a similar situation in the future. It is a false statements that you *never* have willpower. Think of times when you *did* use willpower. Next determine what you can do the next time you are at your cousin's house for dinner, to avoid eating food you don't want. Write this self-dialogue in your journal.

Repeat this disputation process with every self-defeating thought, until rational thinking becomes second nature. For example, you might think, "Ok, I did eat a piece of cake I hadn't planned to eat, but most of the time I *am* able to stick to my diet (non-permanent). My cousin has a pretty forceful personality (non-personal) and it is hard for anyone to resist her. The next time I am invited to dinner at her house, I will call in advance and tell her that my doctor ordered me to cut out sugar for my health. This way she won't be offended when I refuse dessert (solution)."

Notice Empowerment

YOU FEEL ENERGIZED AND EMPOWERED (E) when you purposefully acknowledge how much better you feel for having purged your mind of defeatist thinking. Write an energizing sentence or two in your journal to reaffirm your new positive perspective. You might write, "I feel much less anxious about going to my cousin's house for dinner. Now I know what to do, and I can do it in a way that doesn't offend her. I will relax and stick to my plan. Even if she does get a little angry I know she will get over it if I emphasize I am doing this for my health".

The ABCDE technique is used to stop cata-strophic thinking and reroute that energy to em-power yourself. The more times you do this, the more automatic the process will become.

Let's reexamine how Myra adds the D and E components to her internal dialogue. Her first step is to dispute (D) her automatic belief that occa-sional overeating is a disaster. Then she determines a plan to do it differently next time. Finally, she reminds herself (E) how the change in thinking makes her feel stronger, and more able to cope with similar situations in the future. The counter-argument rescues Myra from her pessimistic think-ing.

Effective counter-arguments are not empty "I can do it" affirmations. For optimism to take root, it must be based in reality, otherwise it is just fantasy. Reasoning with yourself enables you to get past upsetting situations so that you can do it better the next time. When Myra chal-

> Reasoning with yourself enables you to defuse your negativity.

lenged her irrational conclusions, she realized how silly it was to think that one goof-up meant she was stuck being overweight forever, or that she was a terrible person.

Next Myra recorded the disputation (D) in her journal. "This is ridiculous. I know I ate too much at the buffet, but that spread was so great it would have tempted anyone. That doesn't mean I am doomed to stay overweight. The next time I go to a buffet, I will find out what the menu is ahead of time and eat a healthy snack in advance so I won't be so hungry and won't be as tempted when I get there."

To get the full power of the ABCDE rational thinking tecnique, it is important to acknowledge (E) the good feeling you get after standing up for yourself. Following the disputation statement in her journal, Myra observes, "What a relief it is to know I have a strategy that will help me cope with buffet situations in the future. I am not a bad person, nor doomed to stay overweight forever." As Myra notices how empowered she feels when she changes the belief (B), minor setbacks lose their ability to send Myra into a tailspin. By using this simple technique, you too, can feel strong, renewed, and self-confident whenever you face a typical weight-loss challenge.

Challenges Ahead

SOMETIMES WE ENCOUNTER PROBLEMS that are relatively easy to resolve; other times it takes a lot of work. Weight-loss falls into the second category. You have to be ready to do what it takes to win the battle once and for all. That includes being willing to *change your mind* to change your weight. There are four common stumbling blocks in weight loss.

Overeating Pitfalls

- Exposure
- Disinhibition
- Pleasing others
- Emotional flux

Exposure to Passion Foods

JUST SEEING A TEMPTING FOOD often elicits an automatic eating response. That is why most weight-loss experts recommend cleaning out your refrigerator and cabinets *before* attempting to lose weight. Get rid of as many temptations as possible, ahead of time. Then be as prepared as you can for encounters with other temptations. For instance, Lucy owns a restaurant and is constantly exposed to temptation. As if that weren't challenging enough, on Wednesday the bakery truck delivers their specialty chewy double chocolate brownies—Lucy's passion food. Every Wednesday Lucy tells herself she will only taste a bite—just to see if they are of the "quality expected." As usual, one bite turns into two, then into a half of a brownie, and so on. By the time she realizes what she has done, she has already eaten three or four brownies.

Lucy tells herself she is a spineless wimp which makes her feels awful about herself. The ABC's of Lucy's cookie eating frenzy would go as follows: The antecedent (A) event was automatically eating at being *exposed* to the brownies. The resulting belief (B) was that she is a spineless wimp. The consequence (C) was she felt like a failure. You can see how important it is to fight right back with the disputation (D) and energization (E).

Lucy challenged (D) the evidence to support her belief that she is a spineless wimp. She identified times when she showed courage and will power and wrote these in her journal. She developed a plan to do errands on Wednesdays so that she was out of the building when the bakery items are delivered. She noticed how empowered (E) she felt when disproving that she was a "failure" and creating a solution to deal the situation in the future. She wrote these empowering thoughts in her journal.

Dis-Inhibition

DISINHIBITION IS A SITUATION THAT TRIGGERS US to eat uncontrollably. For some it might be taking that first bite of our favorite "off-limits" food. For others, drinking alcohol is a disinhibitor when trying to lose weight. For example, when Mark takes clients to lunch he drinks a glass or two of wine. He can't understand why he is not taking weight off as quickly as some of his friends, who are following the same diet as he. What Mark doesn't realize is that not only is wine fattening but once he drinks a glass or two, he munches non-stop in social settings. Alcohol makes dieting more difficult, and Mark feels frustrated. He is thinking of throwing the diet "out the window".

> Be prepared for encounters with passion foods.

Here are the ABC's of Mark's disinhibition situation. The antecedent (A) is social drinking, which leads him to overeat. He believes (B) there must be something wrong with him because he doesn't lose weight, while his friends seem to do so without problems. Mark feels depressed (C), and is considering foregoing his diet altogether. Instead, he disputes (D) the erroneous belief that there is something wrong with him for not being able to lose weight. He identifies the fact that he eats uncontrollably when he drinks. He develops a plan to avoid the disinhibitor by ordering non-alcoholic drinks when taking clients to lunch. He feels energized (E) because he identified the problem, and figured out a solution.

Pleasing Others

SOMETIMES WE EAT JUST TO PLEASE OTHERS. Maybe you grew up in a household where food was equated with love and refusing a second helping was equivalent to saying "I refuse your love". We all want to be liked, but we would never agree to drink poison just to avoid hurting someone's feelings. Yet, we agree to eat extra fatty, sugary, or fried foods, which can be poisonous to our health!

Just as we eat to please others, we might try to lose weight for others. In reality, eating and losing weight should be under no one's control but your own. When we give that control away to others we are letting *them* determine what becomes of our body, our health, and our emotions. For instance, Marge's husband is embarrassed to be seen with her because she is overweight. He

> When you give control to others, they determine what becomes of your body.

told her that if she gained any more weight she could move into another bedroom because he did not find her attractive anymore. Marge agreed to lose weight and refrains from eating—in front of her husband. However, she sneaks out of the house and gorges on candy bars and milk shakes. As the scale goes up, so does her anxiety level. *You cannot lose weight for anyone but yourself.*

The antecedent (A) in this example is Marge's husband communicating his disdain for her weight. Her belief (B) is that she should be able to lose weight for him. But she eats in secret, and the scale keeps going up. As a result (C) Marge feels anxious and worse than ever about her weight.

Marge used her ABC's to regain control of her thinking. She pulled out her journal and made the following entry. "I wasn't able to loose weight for Henry, but that doesn't mean I shouldn't try to lose weight for me. Tomorrow I'm going to make an appointment with my doctor (D) to talk over the medical benefits of my losing weight, and I will ask her to give me some small dietary modifications I can try. I feel much better now. (E) If I decide to lose weight after hearing what the doctor tells me, I will do so on my own terms. I will tell Harry I am doing this for me, and I will be doing it my own way. I feel like I'm regaining control over my life!

Emotional flux

ANYONE CAN FALL VICTIM TO MOOD EATING. We eat when we are happy. We eat when we are sad, stressed, depressed, angry, or anxious. We eat when we feel bored, or lonely. Eating in response to emotion instead of physical hunger makes us fat, because it piles on extra calories that our body doesn't need. Mood eating is overcome by becoming aware of emotions that trigger your eating. List these in your journal. Then identify non-food related ways to address your feelings.

Lisa for example, has two small children and works from home. There are days when she can't seem to get a thing done. The stress of trying to run a professional business while the kids are tugging on her, or screaming at each other, often leads Lisa straight to the cookie jar—which she keeps for the kids! Lisa hasn't lost all of her weight from her last pregnancy and worries that with the 12 pounds she gained since the birth that she is beyond hope and doomed to be fat forever. She feels fat and sloppy, yet everyday the same cycle continues.

The antecedent (A) for Lisa' eating is the stressful everyday situation of trying to care for the kids and the business contemporaneously. So Lisa eats to relieve her stress. The stress-eating cycle has become automatic and Lisa believes (B) that she might be beyond hope, so she concludes (C) that she is doomed to be fat.

When Lisa catches herself thinking in this self-defeating way, she pulls out her journal, and disputes (D) her negative thoughts. She writes:

> *"Just because this has happened to me regularly since I started working from home, doesn't mean it has to continue this way. I can reduce stress by scheduling an hour or two to devote to calling clients without interruption. I will hire a high school girl to watch the kids in the other room during those hours. Another plan is to do something other than eating when I am stressed. I will do 12 jumping jacks whenever I feel the urge to head to the cupboard for food."*

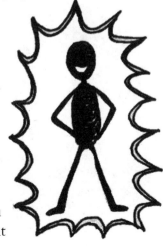

To finish, Lisa will actively energize herself (E) by writing a couple of sentences about feeling hopeful once again, instead of helpless.

Dispute irrational thoughts you tell yourself. Openly argue with them—do it with conviction! Remember, the journal you are keeping is an important component to your success. Document all that you eat, all of the exercise you do, and your emotional reactions throughout the day as you follow your program. Make sure to document your self-arguments, too.

Use the ABCDE method whenever you run into difficulty with your weight-loss plan. Write the steps out in your journal, so that you can refer to them when you face similar situations as you go along. Having a plan

Use the ABC—DE method when you run into difficulty.

and talking back to negativity will enable you to take immediate action in the face of setback. Observe which negative, irrational beliefs make you feel defeated, then figure out ways to challenge them—and win! *Change your mind to change your weight!*

9

Resisting Temptation

HAVE YOU EVER WISHED you could get all food out of the house until you reach your goal weight? Dream on! Fasting is neither healthy nor desirable in most cases. It is healthier to learn to eat in a way that doesn't cause you to gain weight. Central is learning how to deal with food-related temptations. Eating can be a pleasant, life-sustaining behavior—when done properly! Your daily diet should include a variety of nutritious foods so your body is satisfied and strong. Then craving for junk food will subside if you stay away from it for a week or two.

Eating for health and fitness is like problem-solving. Eighty-five percent of problem-solving depends on pre-planning; the other 15 percent depends on having the specific skills required to solve the problem. Here are some common eating-related dilemmas, along with sure-fire strategies for solving them. It is time to roll up your sleeves and get to work!

Day 3 Dilemma

WE ARE ENTHUSIASTIC IN THE FIRST FEW DAYS of starting a new weight-loss program. When the newness wears off, reality sets in and we begin to crave the foods we have cut out. Around the third or fourth day, we become bored, or frustrated, and all heck breaks loose! We may not only chuck the weight-loss plan, but also start to eat more than we would have if we hadn't begun to diet in the first place! To stay motivated, develop a plan for when you reach the *day three dilemma*. Of course for some of us it happens on day 5, or week 4 or month 3. Eventually we all reach a point in which motivation ebbs. How can we avoid jumping ship when the newness wears off?

Old is New Again Technique

THE SOLUTION to heading off the Day 3 Dilemma is to select a weight-loss and exercise program that allows enough flexibility to vary your menus and exercise techniques, while still staying within the limits of the program.

When you start to feel bored or frustrated, review your program in writing in your journal. Think of small ways to give it a new twist. Figure out how many modifications you can make to your current routine to keep yourself motivated. For instance, instead of speed-walking all the time, try interval walking–alternating fast and slower paces. Instead of preparing your supper at home every night, go to a restaurant that accommodates your weight-loss requirements. Instead of eating the same fruit everyday, incorporate new fruits that are permissible on your program. Making occasional changes to your program lends new excitement to your journey; making it less likely you will get bored and give up.

Special Occasions

WE TYPICALLY EAT MORE on special occasions— birthday parties, christenings, or co-worker's retirement celebrations. Excuses to celebrate and overeat pop out of the woodwork. A friend of mine once sighed, "There must be a way we can go to all of these celebrations and avoid overeating and gaining weight—after all they are a part of life! There absolutely is a way we can do this. It is called the *It's My Party and I'll Slim Down if I Want to Technique.*

It's My Party Technique

THE TRICK IS TO TAKE OUT YOUR JOURNAL and plan out your party-going strategies *ahead of time*. Decide what you will eat and drink and then stick to the guidelines you set for yourself. Pride comes from being able to resist what you know looks good on the surface, but will do you harm in the long run. Focus on getting your warm fuzzies through great conversation, and not through eating extra food. People, not potato chips are the real reason for the occasion.

Let's face it. We spend billions of dollars a year on weight loss products, and ignore the one method that works—eat less, exercise more. You

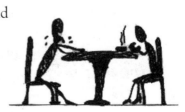

can't abandon this guideline whenever a special
_____ occasion arises, and expect to stay fit

Start with one
small change. and trim. It is important to learn to
work through temptations at special
occasions, so that you can continue to
live life fully, without feeling deprived. The real
celebration is your healthy, fit body.

Start by making only one small change at a
time. For example, at buffets fill your plate only
once. Practice this at the next event. Then add
another small change to your usual buffet routine—
avoid dishes swiming in butter or mayonnaise.
Plan these changes out before every social event you
attend; adding small additional changes each time.
In your journal, pre-plan how much you will eat,
what you will do at the party when you are not
eating, and what you will do for physical activity
before hand, to make up for some special foods
you will allow yourself, beyond your daily food
allotment.

Aunt Josie Dilemma

EVERYONE HAS AN AUNT JOSIE. Her name might be

Don't be pressured
into eating food you
don't want. Just say
"No!" again, and
again, and again.

Jane or Millie, but you know
deep down who she is. She is
pushy and insists that you eat a
piece of her blueberry pie. You
don't want the pie, but you
don't want to offend Aunt Josie
even more. Offending her would
be unpatriotic! There is only
one way to avoid being pressured into eating food
that you don't want.

Broken Record Technique

THE BROKEN RECORD TECHNIQUE simple and powerful. While remaining calm, firmly repeat, "No thank-you" again and again until the other person *hears* it. Keep your voice mild and your tone respectful. That's all it takes. When someone insists you eat against your will, remind yourself that only *you* have a right to determine what you eat. You can be assertive without being aggressive or offensive and people will eventually understand that you mean business. After all, your health is at stake!

10

More Temptation Stoppers

DINING OUT CAN BE THE DOWNFALL of even the most saintly dieters. We may have been sailing along with our program for weeks. Our homes are safely stocked with the appropriate nutritious foods. We have reeducated ourselves about portion control. We have surrounded ourselves with supportive people. All in all, we have no problems sticking with our diet when we are in our own home or office environment.

Now you have to leave your safety net. Some old college buddies contact you about a get-together at one of the best Italian restaurants around—and Italian food happens to be your favorite! You haven't seen these folks for several years and you'd really like to go—but how are you going to handle all of that temptation without feeling either deprived or out of control? One option is to use the Roadmap!

Roadmap Technique

YOU WOULD PROBABLY NEVER THINK of taking a trip without knowing exactly where to go, how to get there, and where to stay once you arrive. You get a roadmap ahead of time and use it to chart your course.

The same approach will help get you where you are going in your new eating adventure. Think of your journal as a roadmap. Before you go to a restaurant, you chart out the waters ahead of time and document them for future use. First, call ahead or stop by the restaurant to see what will be on the menu. Then plan and write down what you will eat and drink—to the last detail. Make a promise to yourself to stick to your plan. Put that promise in writing. You are less likely to break a written contract with yourself.

Common disasters-in-waiting include the bread basket, alcoholic beverages, large portion sizes, endless choices, the butter and cream sauces—and of course, the social setting itself. Eating in company disinhibits our ability to limit our eating. We tend to get carried away with the good feeling that comes with conviviality and forget about our resolve to eat sensibly. Be alert for this danger and make no exceptions regarding staying true to your diet and exercise plans. Losing weight is hard enough. Don't sabotage your efforts by convincing yourself that this one time doesn't count. *Every time counts.* In the end, all of the "isolated" occasions add up. Be prepared for these feelings in advance. Imagine them vividly in your mind and see yourself reacting to them with strong resolve.

Detail Your Itinerary

THE TRICK IS TO MAP OUT A DETAILED ITINERARY for yourself that will take you smoothly from point A, your home, to point B, the restaurant and safely back home again. Planning ahead of time helps to avoid feeling either deprived or overindulgent. You will know what to order before you look at the menu. You will be prepared to push away the breadbasket so it won't tempt you. You will order seltzer with just a spritz of wine instead of a full glass of wine or other alcohol, which makes you lose track of how much food you eat. You may decide to split the portion in your plate before beginning your meal and take the rest home for tomorrow's lunch. That's not only slimming, but cost-effective, too!

Visualize Success

TAKE A FEW MINUTES TO VISUALIZE being with your friends around the restaurant table. See yourself enjoying the company and conversation, without putting fork to mouth the whole time. See yourself sitting with a cup of coffee or tea after your meal while catching up on old times. Remind yourself that the real joy is in the company, not the calories.

> Mentally rehearse exactly what you will do when faced with temptation.

Restaurant eating doesn't have to be a source of anxiety. Change your mind, and think of restaurants as pleasant challenges, instead eating frenzies waiting to happen. You will come home from your "trip" safely, feeling refreshed, and renewed. Bon voyage!

Just do It technique

SOMETIMES THE GOING SIMPLY GETS TOO ROUGH on our journey to fitness. Temptation, laziness, and lack of motivation seem a lot stronger than we are. Decisions are made in a split second during these times, and it is just as easy to make a right one, as it is a wrong one. These are times when you just do it anyway—using the sheer force of willpower. Willpower is not a dirty word. It connotes strength. There are some things we must do to safeguard our health without stopping to debate about it. Don't ruminate about how unfair this is. Instead, take pride in doing hard work, knowing you will achieve lasting and meaningful results. Think of self-discipline as the guardrail along the highway to self-esteem.

Beth and her husband Lyle, for example, started a weight-loss program but the insidious availability of snack foods made it seem impossible. "Temptations are all over the place", wailed Beth. "At work there was a big tray of mixed nuts on the table. The other day someone had a birthday and there was a cake from the pastry store on the desk next to mine. Lyle isn't doing much better either!" Lyle's problem was the junk food at home. "Those twink-dogs that Beth buys for the kids seem to have my name on them," he whined.

Beth and Lyle sounded like helpless victims of Madame Food the Dominatrix! We can't avoid temptations—they are a reality of life. There isn't always time to plot out a new motivational strategy in your journal. Sometimes you forget to get the twink-dogs out of sight so you won't be tempted to gobble them down. You can, however, call upon your inner strength and power. Just trust that it will be there when you need it. You may not *want* to pass on that piece of cake. Just *do it anyway* while telling yourself that you will not give temptation the power to unravel you and weaken your resolve to reach your goal.

Dieters are often convinced they are "victims". They see themselves as victims of metabolism, victims of an evil fast-food culture, and victims of well-meaning mothers who force three portions their cooking on them. It is easy to believe that everyone and everything has control over us. The truth is, you are strong. You don't need to be shielded from doughnuts and pizza for the rest of your life. Nor do you need to be carted off to a psychotherapist to get over every "unplanned for" bowl of peanuts! There is a more efficient and empowering solution: Your ability to think rationally.

As children we had trouble delaying gratification. Now we are wiser and stronger. Even if tempting foods are all around, so what? That's life. Refuse it. How? Just do it! Remind yourself that there is something you want that is more important and longer lasting than a brief taste of chocolate.

The more times you refuse to eat greasy fries out of sheer willpower, the less effort it will take to do so next time. It takes about 6 weeks to form a solid new habit. Just keep "doing it" one day at a time and you *will* be able to eliminate free-form snacking. No matter what the late-night infomercials tell you, you *can't* snack all day long and lose weight. Tell yourself, " I may not like this, but I'm tough and I will *do it anyway*." Little by little the temptation will lose its strength.

Bella Figura Technique

WHEN WE DON'T LIKE OUR BODIES we often let our appearance deteriorate. Then we look in the mirror and our neglected appearance makes us like ourselves even less! There is a definite connection between how we look and how we feel about ourselves.   In Italy, the cultural phenomenon of *bella figura* is the common practice of putting your best foot forward in how you carry yourself and how you present yourself. Take time for grooming, like the Italians do, to whom beauty depends neither on money nor perfect physical attributes. What matters is how you feel about yourself. If you feel you have been letting your appearance go, make a point to invest time in *you*. Play up your good features and admire them in the mirror. When you *think* "attractive" you will *become* more attractive.   Making a habit of doing things to improve how you feel about your appearance will have big payoffs in terms of our psychological well-being

> When you think "attractive" you become attractive.

Feel Good, Look Good

DON'T CONCENTRATE on outside appearance only, take care of your inside appearance as well.   Replace negative self-statements with solutions, regarding your appearance. When you notice you are telling yourself you are unattractive, remind yourself of your attractive features. Everyone has least one feature that they like about ourselves. Start with that! Instead of telling yourself, "I look like a blimp in this shirt", find a solution—such as changing into a shirt that you do like.   Then make sure to tell yourself how great you look! Make personal appearance important, but don't obsess about it. In addition to getting trimmer, you will look better and feel more confident. Write about your appearance dilemmas and how you will solve them in your journal. You will feel better about yourself right away instead of having to wait until you have lost weight.

Thought Stoppng Technique

SOMETIMES WE TAKE JUST ONE BITE and then can't seem to stop eating. Sometimes the uncontrollable urge to binge-eat comes when we have deprived ourselves. It can also happen when we let ourselves get too hungry, or after a couple of alcoholic drinks. If you frequently eat to the point of discomfort, you should have a talk with your physician, who will help you determine if you are suffering from an eating disorder. Most of us simply have milder cases of uncontrolled eating which center around our trigger foods—foods that we have a hard time resisting.

Even with the best laid plan you may still fall prey to uncontrollable eating sprees. An effective technique for stopping an overeating episode—before it starts, or in midstream—is called *Stop Thought*. Here's how it works. When you are tempted to overeat or even while you are in the process of overeating suddenly shout "Stop!", and picture a big red stop sign. Hearing "Stop!" is like a wake-up call that brings what we are doing into consciousness. The best part is, it doesn't matter at which point you find yourself in the over-eating cycle. Stopping *always* makes sense!

Don't shout the word "Stop!" out loud if you are in company. It is enough to shout it silently to yourself, then distract yourself with another activity immediately. Always substitute one behavior for another or you are likely to go right back to the negative behavior you were trying to replace. Put on some relaxing music, for example. Put a stick of sugarless chewing gum in your mouth. Go and make the acquaintance of someone new in the cafeteria. Get out and take a walk around the block during the coffee break. Do five jumping jacks. *Do something,* anything that is positive, and contributes to your fitness goals.

Check negativity at the dook.

11
EXERCISE

HERE IS NO FREE RIDE. Magic pills are myth—including the one that I saw advertised on TV, called Exercise in a Jar. We've all fallen for such nonsense at one time or another. My friend was promised astonishing results after wearing special shorts for only an hour a day for two weeks. All the weight George "lost" from wearing the shorts, reappeared as he drank water. Deep down, we all know that we have to sweat and breathe heavily to get into shape. There is no magic pill.

Put in the Effort

REGULAR EXERCISE MAKES IT EASIER to take weight off and keep it off. Exercise does *not* come in a jar. You've got to put out the effort. Research shows that exercise has important effects on psychological well-being, too. Imagine how confident you will feel when you start to notice those nicely shaped muscles, that invigorating feeling and rosy glow on your skin after a good aerobic workout. Regular exercise helps ward off depression and negativity, making it easier to maintain a positive outlook on life. Regular exercise boosts self-esteem and fills our brains with those feel-good brain chemicals that make us want to say "yes" to the day ahead! The evidence indicates that adults suffering from chronic health problems, such as high blood pressure or heart disease, can lower their short-term risk of death by exercising for as little as 30 minutes a week. That's the power of exercise!

Exercising Specifics

WORK WITH YOUR DOCTOR to determine your exercise guidelines. The U.S. Department of Agriculture Dietary Guidelines and the National Heart, Lung, and Blood Institute's (NHLBI) Clinical Guidelines recommend decreasing calories and engaging in at least 30 minutes or more of moderate physical activity on most days of the week. Unfortunately, only 22 percent of men and 19 percent of women follow these guidelines—even though it directly improves the quality of life! In your journal, write down a list of exercise possibilities that appeal to you, then share them with your doctor and discuss safe exercise guidelines for *your* body

Right Activities for You

MAKE SURE TO INCLUDE ACTIVITIES that you *enjoy* doing. If you hate playing tennis under the hot sun, go swimming instead. If bicycling hurts your bottom, try brisk walking. Do what you enjoy and keep track of your results in your journal. This will give you instant ammunition when you face an exercise slump.

Try different activities and observe your reactions to them. Write down the time of day that you exercise, and the type of exercise you do. Then write a few words pertaining to your thoughts about that exercise session. Be honest! If you had an unpleasant experience analyze what caused it. Perhaps 7AM is too early for your body clock, for example. A lifetime of physical fitness requires a lifetime of staying active. Make sure there is variety in your exercise routine. You can alternate between weight-lifting sessions, aerobics, stretching, and Yoga, for example.

Lifestyle Activities

INCREASE YOUR OVERALL DAILY ACTIVITY so you burn even more calories throughout the day. Being constantly on the move puts your metabolism in a weight-loss mode. For example, you could take the stairs instead of the elevator, park your car in the farthest available space, or walk to the mailbox instead of driving. Make three or four trips down to the cellar to wash the laundry, instead of using the laundry chute. Walk around the block during lunch hour, instead of hanging out with coworkers in the cafeteria. Small changes such as these will make a huge difference in expending more calories.

A lifetime of fitness requires a lifetime of being active.

Variety

EXERCISE SHOULD NEITHER BE PAINFUL, nor so vigorous that it leaves you gasping for air. If you are experiencing pain, change your way of exercising! You won't stick with something that requires a superhuman sacrifice. On the other hand, don't let normal soreness or stiffness stop you from exercising. The reason that "workouts" are so named is because it takes work to lose weight. When fighting the battle of the bulge, be armed! Your best ammunition is to have a variety of exercises ready to be deployed, should one or the other not work out for you. Think of exercise as a never-ending adventure. Try lots of different activities. As long as you keep moving, you'll get there. The problem with skipping a day—especially if you are just starting an exercise program—is that it becomes much harder to start again. Be prepared with a plan to overcome this and get back to exercising. A

> You won't stick to a program that requires super-human sacrifice. So don't try!

body in motion stays in motion, so keep the momentum going!

If your muscles nag you the day after you lift weights, don't panic. A bit of muscle soreness is perfectly normal and means your muscles have been stimulated in a healthy way. When you feel sore one day from using certain muscle groups, simply choose another type of activity for the next day.

Moderation

IF YOU ARE FEELING WEAK OR TIRED most days after exercising, determine if your routine is too vigorous. Make sure you are eating a variety of nutrient-rich foods that are low in fat and high in energy-promoting nutrients. You should be getting *at least* 1200-1500 calories if you are a woman, and 1800-2000 calories if you are a man. Your weight-loss plan should never suck the life out of you. If it does, you may not be consuming enough calories, or enough nutrients, or you may be exercising too vigorously.

Modify your eating or exercise routines when you feel it is necessary. Your eating plan should leave you energized and feeling better than ever while losing weight at a slow pace. Never go to extremes in eating or exercising. The objective is to acquire long-lasting healthful behaviors that you can follow for a lifetime.

You can make certain trigger foods "off limits" while in the process of losing weight. Alternatively, you may decide to learn to eat passion foods in moderation, without going berserk. The *moderation* approach takes preplanning. List in your journal which foods you will eat and the amount, without going off of your weight-loss plan.

If you choose the *abstinence* approach, you may face a couple of tough weeks at first until your desire for that food eventually decreases. Aversive imagery can help. If your trigger food is chocolate chip cookies, for instance, you might imagine that the cookies are ant-infested, so you will no longer want to eat them.

Rainy-Day Plan

RAIN? SNOW? SLEET? That's precisely why they invented exercise equip-

ment, videotapes, and indoor malls!
Don't let bad weather turn you into
an exercise dropout. Empower
yourself with alternatives and you
will arrive at your destination.

Yoga gives the
body a stretch and
calms the mind.

When bad weather tries to defeat you, get back up
fighting. Write out an alternative plan in your
journal ahead of time, so you will be prepared. On
rainy days you might try mall-walking, lifting light
hand weights at home, or plugging in that exercise
videotape and getting your body moving in the
comfort of your own living room. Setting a regular
time for exercise each day will turn doing it into a
habit, and nothing else will take precedence.

For even more motivation on rainy days, save
something special for the occasion. Try something
new—like a power yoga class or tape. Yoga is become hotter than ever, because it not only gives
your body a great stretch, but also
calms your mind—indispensable when
in the process of trying to lose
weight!   Power or Asthanga yoga
builds heat in the body. It is
both aerobic and anaerobic, so
that all of your muscles are
worked, including the most important one—your heart.

Bargain News

WIPE OUT ALL EXCUSES NOT TO EXERCISE. If money is
a problem, don't worry. Exercise need not cost you
a dime beyond a good pair of gym shoes. Walking
and running are free activities. If weight training is
your thing, you don't need a fancy, expensive gym.
Russell, for example, thought he might have to stop
exercising when his gym membership ran out. It

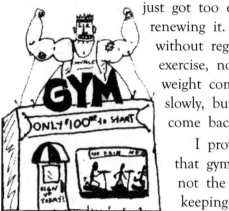

just got too expensive to keep renewing it. Yet he knew that without regular physical exercise, not only did his weight come off more slowly, but it would also come back more quickly!

I proved to Russell that gym memberships are not the only option for keeping those muscles in shape. Another option is in the free bargain newspaper. Even the daily local newspaper offers a variety of ads for weights, aerobic machines, and other kinds of fitness equipment. Some of it is in great condition—just make sure you check it out in person before you agree to lay out your money. Sometimes exercise equipment will be offered free, in exchange for removing it from someone's house! Now get going—the world really is at your fingertips!

Simple Wisdom

Student to Fitness Guru: Tell me, which exercises really work? I don't want to waste my time.

Fitness Guru to Student: The only exercise that works, is the one you do.

ImPRESS Yourself!

GETTING AND STAYING MOTIVATED can be difficult when it comes to exercise. Henry Murray, the originator of Needs Theory, in psychology, believed that behavior is the result of two forces—needs and press. *Needs*, our internal drives, make us respond in a certain way, under certain conditions. There are biological needs and psychological needs. We have a biological need to eat, for example. We have a psychological need to socialize. *Press* is the other half of what motivates our actions. They are the objects, situations, and events—or our interpretation of those events—that goad us to take action towards fulfilling our needs. If I am hungry—*need*—and food is in front of me—*press*, I will eat.

Needs and press can provide important motivational weight-loss tools when we learn how to adjust them a bit. For example, if you can't seem to get exercising, take your journal out and convince yourself why you *need* to exercise. Find evidence to affirm this need. You might research the latest information about the benefits of exercise. If there is heart disease somewhere in your family line, for example, find information on how exercise benefits and prevents heart conditions. Start with the issues that are important to you, and find arguments that will increase your need to work out.

Next, work on your press. Set up your environment so that it is conducive to working out. For instance, have your exercise equipment easily within reach, or have a date set up with a walking buddy, which you can't back out of. In other words, im*press* yourself!

When you develop a strong need to exercise and your surroundings put pressure on you or *press* you to do so, you will be much less likely to skip an exercise session. Manipulate both your needs and press so that skipping the exercise session is not an option.

12

READY, SETBACK, GO!

O BSTACLES, DIFFICULTIES, MOMENTARY SLIP-UPS, and perceived failure, are all part of life. What do Bill Clinton, Donald Trump, Richard Nixon, Thomas Edison, and Michael Jordan have in common? All of them seem to have an unparalleled ability to rebound from difficulty. Each knew what it was like to fail, then pick themselves up again and keep plugging away until they succeeded.

Achieving your fitness goals is the same as accomplishing anything else in life. Persistence and elbow grease separate the winners from the losers. How you cope with setback determines how resilient and persistent you will be in reaching your goals. What you say to yourself when you experience setback is more important to your success than genetics, intelligence, or natural ability.

Psychologist Benjamin Bloom studied high achievers in the fields of sculpting, Olympic swimming, tennis, mathematics, music, and research. What he found was that drive and determination—not inborn natural talent—is often the deciding factor for success. One's style of coping with "failure" is what separates optimists from pessimists, and thus winners from losers. Remember, optimists explain disappointment as *temporary, specific* and *non-personal*. It also helps to be thoroughly convinced that the goal you are working towards is right for you. Getting fit will improve your physical and mental well-being, but you have to *want* these benefits in order to be able to work through the tough times.

The real challenge is keeping the weight off.

Losing weight is hard but almost any sound diet and exercise plan will work. *Keeping* the weight off can be the real challenge. A survey by the Calorie Control Council Consumer Survey found we have difficulty maintaining our weight because we make the following common mistakes: don't exercise enough; splurge too often on favorite foods; eat too many high fat foods; eat for emotional reasons; overeat at mealtimes; eat improperly at restaurants; watch only fat, not calories; watch only calories, not fat. To which of these errors do you succumb? Write them down. Think of past weigh-loss efforts and the situations, people, and things (e.g., certain foods) that made it hard for you to stick with your weight-loss program. For example, are television commercials your downfall? How about seeing certain foods that you love? Do you overeat when you are in the company of certain people? Are there particular social events that lead to free-for-all eating? Write all of these down while they are fresh in your mind.

Prepare for Setbacks

BE PREPARED FOR SETBACKS AND RELAPSES. They happen to all of us. Once you identify your high-risk situations—situations that cause you to break your diet or exercise commitment to yourself—list them in your journal and develop a strategy to use to combat each. For example, you might realize that you overeat when you have salty snack foods in the house and when your boss gets you angry. Don't buy the chips and pretzels in the first place. Substitute a quick walk around the workplace for eating when you feel frustrated with your boss.

Write out your plan for counteracting set-backs when you are in a calm, rational frame of mind. Don't wait until you are in the middle of a setback and upset. Your plan should deal with specific strategies and self-arguments to combat high-risk situations. The more information you put into your journal now, the more efficiently it will guide you when you need it later on.

Small weight-gains are easier to reverse than are large gains.

Monitoring your weight on a weekly basis is a good habit because it is much easier to reverse small weight gains—as a result of a few slip-ups—than it is to reverse larger weight gains of ten or twenty pounds. Studies show that those who are successful at loosing weight and keeping it off take control over small weight gains and have a plan to reverse the extra poundage right away.

Common Excuses

IT IS HUMAN NATURE TO JUSTIFY what we do, even if what we are doing is not good for us. We all come up with excuses that absolve our consciences of weight-loss wrongdong. For example, we might think that we deserved to eat that extra helping of dessert because we just got a promotion. Or perhaps we felt a bit sad today and decided to pamper ourselves by watching TV all day and foregoing the exercise. And of course, we know how upset Mom gets if we refuse a big slice of her chocolate cake. Who could disobey Mother? The trouble that one excuse leads to another, then to another while one regained pound leads to five. Get serious about losing weight. Tell yourself point-blank—**no more excuses!** Here are some ideas for conquering common excuses to justify foregoing your program.

It's the Kids

IT IS DIFFICULT TO GO OUT RUNNING when you have no one to watch the kids. Be creative in your solutions and you will come up with something suitable for your lifestyle and your wallet. You might take one kid in the baby pack and push the other in the stroller. Better yet, get a jogging stroller—the best piece of baby equipment ever invented. Babies love the motion and you get a great workout to boot!

If your kids are a bit older, take them on a walking path and let them ride their tricycles while you power walk alongside them. There are plenty of sports activities you can
do with your
little ones
that don't
cost a lot of
money—like
volley ball,

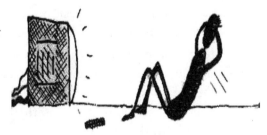

badminton or a good game of basketball in the driveway. Such simple activities bring you and your family closer together, while you keep the pounds off.

I Can't Resist Sugar

WE ONCE THOUGHT that sugar consumption was benign except for the threat of dental cavities. Now research suggests that excess sugar may contribute to adult onset diabetes, obesity, and even loss of vitality of the skin and hair. Sugar also has an addictive quality, making it nearly impossible to stop eating. If this is true for you, you would do better to stay away from sugar completely, similar to a former alcoholic would stay away from liquor or a former smoker would avoid cigarettes.

Begin by making the commitment to go without sugar and sugar products for a several days, until the craving subsides. There will be moments in which you will feel like you will never make it, but eventually your "addiction" to sweets will wane and disappear if you stay tough and determined to succeed. If sugar is the reason you are overweight, it may be necessary to eliminate it completely. Many times this works better than trying to moderate sugar intake. When you have reached your goal weight, you can always decide if you want to reintegrate sweets into your diet on an occasional basis, such as on special occasions, or continue to stay away from sugary foods altogether.

There are some very tasty sugarless dessert recipes available. Some use healthy sugar substitutes, such as fruit puree', fructose, brown rice syrup, or stevia. Experiment with some of these alternatives to see if they work for you.

I Love High-Fat Foods

IF YOU EAT A LOT OF FRENCH FRIES, chips, ice cream, red meat, and pizza, you are probably taking in too many calories from fat. Check the labels. Make sure that each portion of the food you are eat contains less than 30% of its calories from fat. Beware of high protein/high fat diets whose long-term effects have been controversial and inconclusive. Make sure your diet plan is healthy, balanced, and contains a wide variety of healthy food choices, small amounts of healthy fats, such as found in fish, olive oil, and flax seeds.

I Eat When Upset

DO YOU EAT WHEN STRESSED, sad, disappointed, excited, happy, angry, anxious, or afraid? If you identify which emotions stimulate you to overeat, you can train yourself to respond to them differently. Instead of overeating in response to stress, for example, substitute relaxation breathing.

Relaxation Breathing

Take a deep breath for a slow count of four, hold it for a slow count of six, and release it for a slow count of seven. Do this two or three times and you will feel both the stress—and the urge to eat—melt away.

Instead of eating in response to sadness, take decisive action to perk yourself up—like putting your favorite CD on and dancing around the living room or by calling a friend who makes you laugh. Make a special section in your journal where you write down which emotions trigger overeating and what responses you can substitute for overeating when you experience them.

I Overeat

TAKE A TIP FROM JOHN TRAVOLTA. When asked how he had pared down for a particular movie role, he pointed to a trick he learned from fashion models. "I eat everything I want", he said, "only I eat less". Portion control is where most of us fall short. We heap the mashed potatoes on our plates and have no idea that in reality, we have piled on 4-5 normal-sized portions.

If you typically put double or triple servings of food on your plate each day and then go back for seconds, you are probably eating double or triple the day's calories! Then you wonder why you are not losing weight! Trimming portion sizes is a painless way to cut calories. Cut your portions down by a third to a half and watch the weight melt off. Chewing your food thoroughly also gives your brain a chance to signal to your stomach that you are full *before* you have eaten too much.

Restaurants Dangers

GOING TO A RESTAURANT CAN WREACK HAVOCK on a weight-loss program. It may be the festive atmosphere, or the array of temptations. One simple technique is to ask the waiter to remove the bread-basket, taco chips, and the Chinese fried noodles from the table. There is nothing more tempting when you are hungry than a bowl of chips and salsa or a basket of sourdough on the table enticing you. Stand your ground, and remind yourself of your commitment to a healthy new body.

Alcohol

ALCOHOL IS ANOTHER TEMPTATION that can be harder to resist when in a restaurant setting. Few realize how fattening alcoholic beverages are. When the waiter asks what you want to drink, order sparkling water with a twist of lime. It looks like a "drink" and is as festive—but without the calories!

Dessert

DESSERT IS A CHALLENGE for even the strongest willed dieters—especially when faced with a tray heaped with luscious selections fit for a queen. If you can't resist, split one. You will get that sweet taste like at the end of a meal without overstuffing yourself on sugar calories. Better yet, ask for fresh fruit. Alternatively, you can end a meal with a cup of coffee or tea and skim milk.

A useful restaurant strategy is to eat only half of your portion. This can be hard to do for those of us who were taught "waste not want not." So we often eat to clear our plates even though we're no longer hungry. But you don't have to feel guilty about wasting food, if you take leftovers home for tomorrow's lunch.

Finally, when dining out, focus your attention on the company and not on food. Eating is more than a momentary sensation on the tongue. It is also a social event that feeds the soul. Savor the wonderful conversation and warm interaction at the restaurant dinner table and you will be less inclined to make food the sole object of your attention.

> Focus your attention on the company, not the food.

I Watch Fat, Not Calories

WE HAVE ALL GOTTEN FATTER since the rise of the low-fat food phenomenon. We were told we could eat cakes, doughnuts, muffins and ice cream—and not have to worry about getting fat as long as we're eating low-fat. What a modern-day miracle! We could eat all of the foods we loved without gaining an ounce. I repeat—there is no magic to losing weight. There is *only* hard work.

Low fat foods replaced their fat content with sugar, which created another dependency. Is there anyone who could really eat one "serving size" of low-fat devil's food cake? The truth is, you must cut out or cut down on your "addictive" foods. Period. The bottom line will always be the same, no matter how you slice the cake. to lose weight, you must burn more calories than you take in.

Watching Calories, Not Fat

WHEN YOU COUNT CALORIES but are not attentive to amount of fat you are taking in, you can compromise your weight and your health. Cut out unhealthy polyunsaturated oils, lard, margarine, and butter. Olive oil, flaxseed oil, and canola oil are good oils. However, oil is still fat and fat is highly caloric. Always use oil sparingly. Unhealthy fats are plentiful in store-bought baked good, so check your food labels for fat content.

13

Rationalize Beliefs

THERE IS A STRONG LINK is between beliefs, emotions, and behaviors. It takes skill to reframe your beliefs to empower, not hinder your goals. Ellis emphasizes that our emotional experience is related to how we think. How we explain what happens to us determines how we feel. When we change our thinking, we can stop setting off the emotions that make us miserable. This is accomplished this by giving more reasonable interpretations to the things that happen to us.

Frequently we interpret negative events in a self-defeating way. In weight-loss, it is important to dispute the negative beliefs that make us miserable after a slip-up. The trick is to interpret slip-ups as temporary, non-personal, and specific. When you are upset, bring your thoughts back into perspective by questioning the evidence that supports your self-defeating beliefs. Then come up with a plan to avoid similar slip ups in the future.

> Interpret slip-ups as temporary, non-personal, and specific.

Get a Grip On Reality

Situation: You ate two pieces of cake and went over your allotted calories for the day.

Self-defeating thinking: I have no willpower (*personal*). I can never resist cake when it is in front of me (*permanent*). I have a hard time denying myself anything (*pervasive*).

Rational thinking: That cake looked so luscious it would have tempted anyone (non-personal). It may have gotten the better of me this time, but I have resisted cake before, and I will do it again (*temporary*). Just because I couldn't resist the cake today, doesn't mean that I have trouble in the future turning down other things I like but are not good for me (*specific*). After this I will make sure there is no cake around in the house (*future plan*).

Discussion: It is important to avoid overdramatizing when you slip up. Calling the situation for what it is, allows you to aoid self-blame and move on with a clear-headed solution.

Argue with Emotions

PEOPLE WHO KNOW HOW TO REVERSE RELAPSES are more likely to lose weight and keep it off. You must cultivate an optimistic attitude—with a realistic twist. The errors we make in life can render us helpless or empower us to forge ahead—it all depends on how we react to them. We all feel lousy when we screw up—that's human nature. Why do some of us rebound while others stay down? Seligman's research indicates that those who feel *helpless* stay down longer. Such people erroneously think that no matter what they do, it won't make a difference. Our reaction to setback—the B-belief part of the ABC paradigm—can empower us or trigger feelings of helpless. Ellis demonstrated that people could gain emotional independence by carefully choosing the thoughts they allow into their heads. Essentially, we create our perspective with the words we use. We can see the glass as

Error can render us helpless or challenge us to forge ahead.

half-full or half-empty. We can believe that a slip-up can blow our whole diet, or we can view slip-ups as something to be expected and begin again. Think like an optimist and you will recover faster from relapse.

Suppose that for the past two days you have been too tired to go for an after dinner walk. Instead of thinking that you blew your exercise regime and losing motivation to exercise, accept that you have fallen into a temporary slump. Then tell yourself that you will break it *right now* by getting out and walking just one block. Do this immediately and you will see how much better you feel. You will probably want to continue walking beyond that one block.

Perhaps you ate a handful of cookies today, and then couldn't stop. Instead of telling yourself you are an awful person who has no will power, put it into perspective. Tell yourself that realistically, everyone has moments where self-control flies out the window and that you are not a bad person for overeating. The next time you are tempted to overeat, plan to wait ten minutes before giving in to the craving. If you still want the forbidden food after ten minutes, you might allow yourself one or two cookies. Most of the time, however, a ten-minute pause is all it takes to make the craving go away.

Suppose you usually head for the refrigerator after having an argument with your spouse. Without giving it a second thought you have eaten an extra meal that was not on your weight-loss plan. Instead of feeling guilty, tell yourself that from now on you will use words, not food to deal with your anger. Even if you don't want to confront your spouse at that moment, don't head for the refrigerator. Instead, go into another room and write your feelings out in your journal. Later after you have calmed down you can think them through rationally. By this time, the urge to raid the refrigerator will have passed.

Use Your Journal

WRITE A DESCRIPTION OF TOUGH SITUATIONS you have faced while trying to stick to your weight-loss plan in your journal. What beliefs were operating at the time? Were they negative or positive? If after a slip-up, you felt guilty, depressed, disappointed, or angry, write this down. Do a little reality testing of those beliefs. Was the slip-up so awful that you should judge yourself as a bad person? Is a handful of extra cookies worth being depressed for a week?

> The way you interpret setbacks determines how you feel about yourself and how quickly to get back on track.

Note how the way you frame your beliefs determines how you end up feeling helpless or empowered after a tough situation. Now, for each of your negative beliefs think of an alternative way of thinking about the situation. Choose new beliefs! Keep these alternative explanations reasonable and upbeat by emphasizing the specific, non-personal, and non-permanent nature of the setback. Emphasize what you *have* been doing right, such as "I did stick to my diet for three days," or "Last night I walked right past that bag of cookies without eating one." Then, come up with a new approach to handle the setback in the future.

The way you interpret weight-loss setbacks has *everything* to do with how long you feel helpless and defeated and how quickly you recover. None of us is immune to the pain of failure. But ultimately we choose our state of mind. A positive state of mind safeguards against long periods of relapse. Remember, the longer you stay discouraged and demoralized the more of a weight gain you will eventually have to reverse. It pays to nip negative thinking in bud!

14
Take Control

NOTHING FEELS BETTER THAN KNOWING we are
stronger than our circumstances. We are
the only ones who should control what
we do and how we think. We *can* resist
temptation. We *can* make choices that are hard to
make. Our inner strength grows each time we make
choices that are aligned with our goals. Each time
you resist the temptation to overeat or under-
exercise; you strengthen your internal control center.
Turning negative beliefs into more positive, rational
explanations is one way to do this. Some other
strategies include aversive imagery, stimulus control,
thought stopping, and reinforcement.

Aversive Imagery

IMAGINING UNPLEASANT IMAGES is a powerful tool for
overcoming food cravings. It's simple. Create an
unpleasant image and pair that image with a food
that typically triggers overeating. Imagining that ants
are crawling in and out of your chocolate chip
cookie will immediately take away your desire to eat
it. Aversive imagery may also help to extend your
life. Here is an example. Some research indicates

that ten percent of cancers in non-smokers is attributed to being overweight. The next time you are tempted to eat a bowl of salty high-fat chips in front of the TV, imagine how that excess fat in your body is feeding cancer cells.

Experts have also found that obese "apple-shaped" women who carry their fat around their middles have a greater risk of developing Type 2 diabetes and heart disease, than do overweight "pear-shaped" women who carry their fat on their hips and thighs. Using this image you could imagine ribbons of slimy abdominal fat creeping up to choke your heart, the next time you reach for seconds at the dinner table. A study reported in the *Journal of the American College of Cardiology* found that immediately after eating a high-fat meal there is a dramatic drop in the elasticity of the arteries. Imagine your arteries turning to gelatin after one of those fast-food jumbo burgers. Get the picture? If you do, you have taken another step closer to reaching your weight-loss goal!

Consider Mary, who had a weakness for spaghetti. She piled it so high on her plate that it looked like a sandcastle—and enjoyed every forkful! Eventually her passion for spaghetti caused her more frustration than happiness as her weight climbed. She asked me for a quick and efficient mental trick that would stop her spaghetti free-for-alls right in their tracks. I suggested that the next time she came face to face with a heap of spaghetti, she should imagine it as a plate of *worms*. The expression on her face turned

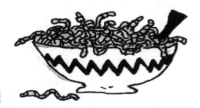

slowly from ecstasy to disgust. "W-o-r-m-s" she exclaimed, "YUK"! That was the point. After a few pairings of something delicious—like spaghetti—with something disgusting—like the image of eating worms—the spaghetti lost its power to trigger uncontrollable eating.

People often ask at which point in the overeating cycle is the aversive-imaging technique most effective. The answer is: At any point! Use aversive imagery before the first bite of your "weakness food". Use it as you are walking over to the cabinet to pull it out. Use it when you have the food in your hand. Use it when you are putting the food to your lips. Reassure yourself that you can stop the overeating cycle at any point in the chain of events. All is not lost after you have taken the first bite!

Stimulus Control

A STIMULUS IS SOMETHING THAT PROMPTS us to feel or act a certain way. Unknowingly, we build strong associations between certain stimuli—like sight, smell, sound, or the thought of something—and certain feelings and actions. The sight of Santa Clause, for example, triggers automatic feelings of excitement. The sound of a song we heard when we were once in love may still trigger nostalgia years later. The smell of a certain dish your grandmother used to make may still conjure up feelings of warmth and security.

The same stimulus-behavior association applies to overeating. For example, if there is a chocolate bar on the table, just the *sight* of it might compel you to eat it. Take away the sight, smell, or thought of the chocolate bar, and you will take away the uncontrollable urge to eat it. The key is to eliminate or limit the stimuli that prompt you to overeat. We all have certain people, places and things in our lives that trigger uncontrolled eating sprees. Start cleaning up your environment to increase your chances of success.

> Remove "eating stimuli" from your environment to increase your chances of success.

Toss out junk food, sugared cereals, and high-fat meats. Respond assertively to people who know how to press your buttons, so you won't need to console yourself with food. Surround yourself and your family with nutritious food and opportunities to exercise. Get the junk foods out of the house. Just the sight of this food is a trigger for eating. Give yourself the gift of breaking unhealthy associations.

You can't surround yourself with your favorite foods then expect not to eat them. Consider Lily whose toxic stimulus was dessert. If it was there, she would eat a couple of portions and then feel anxious about it afterwards. Lily decided to keep desserts away from the dinner table and to substitute healthful desserts, such as fruit. For a few evenings when dessert time rolled around she felt twinges of "withdrawal" but eventually she created new associations to signal the end of mealtime. In addition to eating a piece of fresh fruit, she drank a cup of coffee or went for a brisk walk around the block after she finished her evening meal.

If watching nightly food commercials is a stimulus that sends you to the refrigerator, break that
"commercial-refrigerator" association by linking
commercial time to something else. Some of my
friends do stretching or jumping jacks during commercials. It is hard to eat doughnuts while doing
jumping jacks!

Rewards

IT IS NO SECRET that rewards increase motivation.
getting a paycheck at the end of the week, has a
lot to do with your getting every morning and
going to work. chances are if the paycheck stopped
coming, you'd stop working. The same holds true
for staying motivated with your weight-loss efforts.
Rewards can be used to strengthen weak behaviors.
For example, if you normally have difficulty asking
the waiter to remove the breadbasket, give yourself
that new scarf you've been wanting as a reward for
following through the next time you eat out and
remember to have the waiter remove the bread.

Write a list of things and activities in your
journal that give you pleasure, joy, happiness, and
fulfillment. Use these as rewards to help you stick
to your diet and exercise program. Make sure these
things are not related to food or would cause you
to gain weight. The idea is to build a customized
list of objects and activities that are not fattening,
too expensive, or harmful. For example, Louise loves
to talk on the phone, but is usually too busy to
keep in touch with friends. On her list of rewards,
she wrote: one-half hour phone call to a friend I
haven't seen in a while. Another example is Bob,
who enjoys listening to flamenco music. On his list
of rewards, he wrote: Purchase the new flamenco

CD by Fury. Maria is a young mom who loves bubble baths, but with three small kids, rarely has time to take one. On her list of rewards, she wrote: One 45-minute bubble bath after kids go to bed.

B.F. Skinner showed that when a pleasant state of affairs follows an action, we are more likely to repeat that action. That is what rewarding yourself does. If Jane typically has a hard time sticking to her exercise program, rewards can help. She decides that if she meets her exercise goal of swimming for 35 minutes today, she will reward herself with a cup of fancy coffee at her favorite café. Chances are she will be more likely to exercise again tomorrow.

On the other hand, we are less likely to repeat actions that are followed by unpleasant consequences—punishment. Mark, who had trouble following his diet on weekends, made a contract with himself to do a half hour of extra yard work on the weekend when he overate during the week. This small punishment quickly put weekend eating right back under his own control.

> Use self-rewards and self-punishment to boost your motivation.

Self-reward and self-punishment are effective strategies for those trying to lose weight. Use whichever reward or punishment works for you. Make sure you acknowledge yourself when you succeed at little things. Take away something you like or do something you don't like, but is good for you anyway, when you flub up.

Tailor rewards

EFFECTIVE REWARDS DON'T HAVE TO COST a dime!
The only criterion for a good reward is that it
should work to keep you on track with your diet
or exercise regime. Buy yourself an inexpensive item
you have been wanting or make free time to do
something you've wanted to do. Don't go overboard
buying yourself items that cost a lot—you may end
up eating out of anxiety!

When you are first forming a new healthy
habit, such as replacing sweets with fruit—or breaking an unhealthy habit, such as eating between
meals—rewards are most effective when used after
each little success. A simple check on a checklist
can serve as an immediate reward. You might keep
a chart, for example, and give yourself a check after
each substitution of fruit for sweets. You can decide
how many checks will earn a certain reward that is
on your rewards list in your journal. For example,
seven checks might earn a new bottle of nail pol-
ish; twenty-five checks might be a night at the
movies. When the new habit is formed, space the
rewards out a bit more. For example, if you have
kept to your eating plan for a whole week you can
give yourself a pedicure on Saturday, or pick something else from your rewards lists
that is proportionate to your ac-
complishment.

Rewards will vary according
to personal preferences. Some
typical rewards for losing weight
might include a facial at the salon;
test-driving a new car; playing cards
with friends; sending a week's worth
of shirts to the dry cleaners; taking

a Yoga class; spending the morning having coffee at a café; organizing a basketball game with friends; or phoning a friend you haven't seen for a while. Look over the reward list in your journal. What would you like add or subtract? Refine your rewards list to make it uniquely yours.

Self Punishment

Effective punishments for overeating or not exercising can include doing chores that you hate doing. Another approach is taking away an activity that you enjoy, such as reading the newspaper after dinner, or foregoing the weekly manicure.

In your journal, list activities that you don't like doing, but that need to be done anyway—such as renting the rug cleaner and scrubbing the carpets, weeding the garden, making a dreaded phone call, washing the car, or shopping for your elderly neighbor. These will serve as "punishments" for going off your diet plan. They also act as deterrents to keep you on your plan.

> When you use doing chores to punish overeating, you are likely to get a lot done while losing weight.

In additional to listing the things you don't like to do, list the things you enjoy doing, such as watching TV after dinner, reading the Sunday morning paper, and so forth. Withholding these pleasantries can serve as punishment and help to get you back on track. Make punishment proportionate to the crime! Eating one extra cookie does not warrant having to clean the carpets of the entire house, whereas eating extra cookies every day for a week might. Decide what works for you. Keep notes on what works and what doesn't work in your journal after each day's entry.

15

Reassess Your Plan

SOME BELIEVE THAT GENETICS ultimately determines a person's weight—therefore diets don't work. Many of us have bought into this misleading message and are now more overweight than ever. To make matters worse, many of us have stopped trying to control our weight altogether. The truth is, following a sensible "diet" and exercise program *does* work. In fact, it is the *only* approach that works reliably.

Certainly heredity influences our physical and psychological destiny to some degree, but it does *not* have the final word. *You do!* Even if your parents were fat and your grandparents were fat, you do *not* have to follow their example. You are not psychologically and physically helpless. You *can* outsmart genetics because your eating and exercise *behaviors* are what ultimately determine your weight. The foundation of any good weight-loss program is a daily continuation of sound eating and exercise habits.

After all, you can feel anyway you want, but if your hand doesn't reach your mouth with the buttered toast you won't gain an extra ounce. When you eat right and exercise regularly you'll lose the weight and no one can stop you—not even your ancestors' genes. Changing your thinking will help you to change your eating habits, and good eating habits lead to greater fitness and health.

Have patience with yourself, and proceed forward, one step at a time. Isolated flub-ups will influence your weight less than will the consistent weeks and months of getting back on track again with your weight loss program. If you don't feel as successful as you would like to be, even after following your program for some time, it might be time to reflect about new ways to make your efforts a success.

Just Do It

IF YOUR WEIGHT CONTROL PROGRAM isn't working the way you had hoped, it may be the wrong program, or perhaps you have not been following it closely enough. If the latter is true, don't blame the program. This is your moment of truth! In reality, you may have not limited your calories enough, or exercised as much as you should have. We're all grown up now and we must just do what we have to do.

We override our preference for taking the easy way out all the time. We "just do it" by getting up early to go to work, when we'd rather sleep in. We "just do it" by staying home to watch the kids when we'd rather be on a desert island somewhere, enjoying the sun. When our dog has an accident on the carpet and we'd rather not have to clean it, we just do it. Similarly, unless you are willing to "just do" what it takes to reach a healthy weight, you won't get there.

Take New Action

DON'T FALL INTO THE "FEEL-SORRY-FOR-ME" mode. Give your mind a new way of thinking—rational optimism. To help you stick to the weight-loss program you chose, take some of the individual aspects of this program and master them, one at a time. You have the ability to work beyond any lack of motivation that your mind tries to trap you with. Afterall, your health is on the line.

You might set up specific times throughout the day to stop and do something healthy for yourself. For example, let's say you want to increase the amount of water you drink each day. In your journal, set the specifics as to when you will drink water, and how much of it you will drink. You might write: "I will drink five 8-ounce glasses of water each day—at 8 am, 10am, 1pm, 3pm, and 5pm. Then write a line or two daily about how you did with that pledge. Perhaps there was one particular hour where you consistently found it difficult to drink the water. Think of how you can work around that. Perhaps you need to be reminded to drink water at that hour, or perhaps changing the hour itself will make the pledge easier to stick to.

When you master a good habit, you will feel energized and want to go on to another. Sometimes it only takes one small change in order to feel a renewed commitment to your weight-loss program.

Customize Goals

REWORK ANY ASPECT OF YOUR PROGRAM that is not working for you. Perhaps you were way out in left field when you promised yourself you could immediately go from being a couch potato to jogging the full length of the track, 5 days a week. Customizing goals allows you to take control. Have realistic expectations for your program, and align your goals with what you *can* do. Walk 20 minutes for 3 days and then increase that to 5 days. Then you can upgrade to 5 days of walking and one of jogging, and so forth.

Start your goals where *you* are and not the other way around. The goals you see in magazines and fitness books are guidelines for the masses. They don't know who you are, where you are in your journey, or what feels right for *you*. Tailor your goals to you, rather than trying to fit yourself into someone else's mold.

> Start your goals where you are at, then inch them along to where you want to be.

Evaluate Success

MANY OF US ARE RELUCTANT to keep track of our weight-loss. Often we don't want to face the truth about our progress, especially if we feel we haven't been as successful as we would like. Yet, taking a long-range look at your weight trend can provide you with the key to figuring out where you need to go from here. When you started changing your mind to change your weight, you wrote a realistic weight goal in your journal.

After you have followed your weight-loss program for a while, review your behaviors—from exercise to eating—and consider what has worked and what hasn't, in terms of the actual weight you have lost thus far. If you have kept a weekly record of your weight changes, turn those numbers into a chart to serve as a visual measure of how you have been doing. Next, review your eating and exercise records.

Note that what has been consistently difficult and consider the reason for the difficulty. Finally, make a new pledge to yourself, and modify your program based on what you have learned from reviewing your journal notes. Here is how Lenore reassessed her program on the basis of the information she gleaned from her weight loss chart, and eating and exercise review.

Weight Chart

ONE WAY TO EVALUATE PROGRESS is to lay the numbers out into a chart. How has your weight varied since you started your program? It should be going steadily in the direction of your goal. Below is Lenore's weight chart after 5 weeks. She weighed herself once each week—on the same day and at the same time—and wrote that number down under the week number.

Lenore's Weight Chart

Week 1	176 lbs
Week 2	175 lbs
Week 3	174 lbs
Week 4	176 lbs
Week 5	175 lbs

Lenore could tell from glancing at this weight chart that something wasn't working. Her weight should have shown a slow but steady decrease from week to week with possible plateaus. Instead her progress is not coming fast enough to keep her motivated.

Review Eating Records

WHEN REEVALUATING YOUR WEIGHT-LOSS PROGRESS, go over your food diary to see if you stayed within your allotted fat/calorie allowance each day. If you find that you frequently exceed your allotted calorie count, then those excess calories are the culprit for the lack of steady progress.

Identify Trigger Points

WE KNOW WHEN WE HAVE BEEN OVEREATING, but to get control of our eating we must uncover the trigger points that goad us to overeat. Once identified, we devise a plan to overcome them. When Lenore checked over her notes she realized that she over-ate when she felt sad. She jotted down a solution to avoid similar slip-ups: "The next time I feel sad, I will call one of my friends."

Lenore also found that she had been eating dessert too frequently and she was also snacking excessively between

> Most of us eat more than we normally would at social events.

supper and bedtime. Her solution was: " I will choose my bedtime snacks from a list of snacks on my diet plan. I will only eat one portion. I will also limit my desserts after supper to twice a week."

A social atmosphere tends to goad us into eating more than we normally would. Lenore found that she ate more food when she was out with friends. Her solution was to plan what to eat ahead of time and to be firm about sticking to that commitment. Many people have difficulty controlling food intake when they drink alcohol. If this is the case for you, a solution might be to avoid alcohol altogether or to plan on eating a limited amount of low-fat pretzels with the drink.

Trigger points for overeating vary from person to person. Certain times of day, such as the 4 o'clock slump, or the sight of desired foods can cause you to eat without thinking.

Reevaluate Your Plan

ALWAYS START WITH THE PREMISE that every weight-loss diet requires work and sacrifice. The diet you choose, however, should fit your lifestyle and flow relatively easily once you get into the routine of it. For example, if you initially chose a plan that involves eating just proteins at one meal and just carbohydrates at another and you have to prepare food for others who refuse to eat this way, it may be too difficult to keep this program up over the long run. When reevaluating your eating plan, ask yourself if it includes the foods you would normally eat anyway; if the meals are relatively simple to prepare; and if the menus satiate your hunger.

Review Exercise Records

DETERMINE IF YOUR EXERCISE ROUTINE has been adequate. If you feel you have not been giving it your best effort, increase the number of days that you exercise each week. Perhaps you need to increase the intensity of your workout. If you have been working with 5-pound weights, now might be the time to purchase a pair of 7 or 8-pound weights. Instead of walking at a normal pace, try fast—walking while pumping your arms, or carrying very light hand weights as you walk.

Another way to give your exercise routing a boost is to add a few minutes to your regular exercise sessions. If you typically walk for 35 minutes each morning, increase it to 40. Maybe the activities you have chosen are boring. If you have been swimming for the past several months, you might add something new, like roller-blading.

Lenore checked her weekly records and found that her strolls around the block were not strenuous enough to be effective aerobic exercise. She decided to power walk which was only a step up in intensity from what she had been used to doing. Although it would be a challenge, she was sure she could keep at it.

Make a New Pledge

EVALUATE THE WEIGHT-LOSS GOAL you initially set. Perhaps it was unrealistic. Don't set yourself up for failure. Sure, you know techniques for bouncing back after setback, but why waste your energy sources on continual rebounding? Instead, set yourself up to *succeed.* When your goals are achievable and realistic, you will accomplish them.

Generally, it is better to set short-range, specific goals, rather than long-range, general weight-loss goals. Because they are closer at hand, small short-range goals are more of a sure shot. Specific goals pertain to the individual actions you must take to reach those goals. One example of a specific action-oriented goal is to exercise for at least 30 minutes today. Another example of a specific action-oriented goal is to refrain from eating in between meals for today. These goals are tangible because there is something specific you must do to reach them. They are also effective, because they are actions you can take immediately, which when strung together lead to the same overall outcome—weight-loss.

Set yourself up to succeed!

If, however, you start out with a goal of losing 25 pounds, it will be hard to stay motivated. Because weight loss depends on a number of variables—including fluctuations in body fluid—those twenty-five pounds may come off quickly or slowly. At times weight-loss will not coincide with your compliance to your weight-loss program. That can be discouraging. Setting goals of concrete action that promote weight-loss rather than just a goal weight is much more effective. If you have performed the behavior, you will feel proud and motivated to continue.

If your goal is losing a specific number of pounds, don't make the final number of pounds be your only goal. It is too long-range and general. Instead, consider setting a realistic, short-range goal of 1.5 to 2 pounds a week. This way your continual progress will motivate you to keep going.

Keep Doing What Works

RULE OF THUMB: If it works, keep doing it. If your present diet and exercise routine are enjoyable and _____ you are slowly but surely losing

RULE OF THUMB: weight, stay with them, even if they
If it works, seem boring. Keep doing what works.
keep doing it. Change only when what you are
_____ doing stops working. You don't have to spin your wheels to get where you want to go. Instead, make small variations in your program to keep it interesting and boost your motivation.

Renew Your Optimism

ROBERT ROSENTHAL RESEARCHED HOW EXPECTATIONS influence behaviors. One hundred students were randomly assigned to one of five math classes. The teachers thought the students were assigned were according to ability, when they were actually randomly assigned to the classes. In other words, there was a mix of ability in each group. Students assigned to the "high ability" class scored higher than those in the "low ability" classes, even though in reality, the groups were of equal ability. How could this be? Self-fulfilling prophecy was at work.

The students performed according to what was expected of them. The teachers, without realizing it, had communicated their expectations to the students in subtle ways—through tone of voice, use of criticism, guidance and body language. This is what happens to you when you tell yourself you will or will not succeed. You will accomplish what you expect.

Demand an explanation from yourself as to *why* you think you won't you succeed. Then argue with yourself until you are convinced that you *will*. Do what it takes. Readjust your goals, change your program, or make your kitchen free of tantalizing foods. Most important, stay positive when evaluating your setbacks, so you can avoid a self-fulfilling prophecy of failure. Argue with yourself until you come up with a solid, action-oriented solution. Here are some fundamental characteristics of optimistic thinking.

> SELF-FULFILLING PROPHECY: You will accomplish what you expect to accomplish.

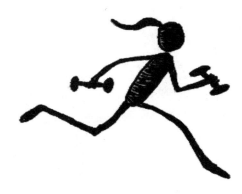

Five Ways to Think Like an Optimist

1. Look at setbacks as temporary, isolated events.
2. Think of setbacks as steps to success.
3. Choose what and how to think.
4. Think in terms of solutions, not problems.
5. Convert negative thoughts into positive ones.

It boils down to choice. Optimism is a *decision* you make, not something that befalls you or that you are born with. People who think optimistically not only enjoy better health and greater self-esteem, but they are also more successful than pessimists in achieving their goals. Once you make optimistic thinking a habit—and it takes about 6-8 weeks to form a new habit—it will be yours forever, to use in all areas of your life whenever you encounter normal predictable setbacks, disappointments, and frustrations.

16
ON YOUR WAY

ATTITUDE CREATES HAPPINESS. Csikszentmihalyi, a foremost researcher on happiness, points out that negative emotions— such as sadness, boredom and anxiety— drain our mental resources, making it hard to cope with life. In contrast, positive emotions liberate our mind, allowing our attention to fully focus on the activity of the moment. Living each moment consciously promotes happiness, inner peace, and freedom from anxiety about the future or the past.

> A happy attitude is the mother of "happiness."

Attitude as Medicine

CSIKSZENTMIHALYI CLAIMS that engaging in activities that we love, that challenge us, and that match our abilities—bring satisfaction and lasting, intrinsic happiness or "flow". Flow is a state of total engagement. One way to love the process of losing weight is to remind yourself of how the process is helping you become stronger, fitter and more vibrant.

Instead of seeing dieting and exercising as dreaded activities, change your attitude, and think of them as exciting challenges. Get excited about the prospect of feeling better and becoming fitter with each effort you make. Learn about your body and the effects of nutrition and exercise on your health. Do everything with enthusiasm and full awareness, even if you don't feel this way on the inside at first. Make every action and thought mean something so that they contribute to a joyful, positive lifestyle. Soon you will feel a sense of pride and "flow" in your daily life. Attitude is everything. Don't associate losing weight with deprivation and suffering. Instead, look at fitness as an exciting challenge that is well-matched to your capabilities. Step up to the plate and swing at the ball!

Make every action and thought mean something.

Expand Your Horizons

BALANCE YOUR LIFE. Don't let weight-loss be the only goal you have. Put your optimism skills into action in *all* areas of your life—especially when you encounter difficult situations. Venture out. Try new things. Develop new interests that take you beyond yourself. Learning new things is a great intrinsic motivator. Think of how many new things there are to get excited about! Have you always wanted to learn how to sail, but never made the time for it? What about that ceramics class you promised yourself you would take, or that yoga studio you wanted to check out? Perhaps you are curious to learn more about comparative religion, foreign politics, or how to write a novel.

Community colleges and adult learning centers offer non-credit courses at very good prices. Why not learn how to roller-blade, ballroom dance, or become proficient in Karate? There is no time like the present. Continuous learning not only keeps your mind fresh, but it enriches your social life, too, as you meet new people who share your interests.

Let yourself become so immersed in your activities that you hardly notice time passing by. Take yourself out of yourself and get engaged with life. This kind of total involvement is the flow. As you learn to get into the flow, you will gradually experience more joy and less negativity. You will berate yourself less. Ruminating about what you don't like about yourself leads to anxiety and depression. Let's face it, everyone can find things they don't like about themselves. Cynthia, for example spends more and more time on her make up and hair, because she feels she never looks quite right. She can hardly pass a mirror without being critical of herself. As a result, she is increasingly depressed, anxious, and has stopped going out with her friends.

Psychologist Aaron Beck who developed cognitive therapy for depression, noticed three recurring themes in the thoughts of depressed patients. The same themes can also be found among people trying to lose weight. They are: a negative interpretation of external events, a pessimistic view of the future, and self-dislike.

To be happy and successful in achieving our goals, it is important to substitute a positive mental attitude for the negative self-statements we automatically fall prey to. Even the most unpleasant situations have a positive side if we look hard enough. Make a game out of finding positive aspects in negative situations. The more you make an effort to reframe your thoughts in a positive way, the more it will become second nature for you to do so. The following table shows how automatic negative interpretations of unpleasant situations can be switched around to their positive counterparts.

Positive Self-Talk

Situation: I had a fight with my wife
> **Negative Self-Statement:** *She gets me so mad I can't talk with her.*
>
> **Positive Alternative:** *Everyone has touchy days. This will pass and then we can talk.*

Situation: I got laid off from my job.
> **Negative Self-Statement:** *I'll never find another job. I will starve.*
>
> **Positive Alternative:** *Sure I'm scared but I can think of this as a challenge. I'll start by getting want ads and sending resumes.*

Sitution: I broke my leg.
> **Negative Self-Statement:** *I can't exercise. I'll never lose this weight.*
>
> **Positive Alternative:** *I can exercise my upper body with light weights from my bed.*

Situation: Edna didn't return my book.
> **Negative Self-Statements:** *That woman never returns anything. She is untrustworthy.*
>
> **Positive Alternative:** *I'll ask Edna for my book. I'll write it out on paper first so I won't be so anxious.*

People who see the glass as half full reach their goals more often. Interestingly, they also have stronger immune systems, and are less likely to get sick than those who see the glass as half empty.

There are three things you can do infuse your daily thoughts with hope, and give yourself an attitude adjustment. First, remind yourself to see the positive aspects of every situation. Next, take some kind of positive action, no matter how small. This will make you feel like you have control of the situation. Finally, find activities you love to do and immerse yourself in them. This will increase your sense of well-being and fortify the cycle of positive thinking.

Optimism Inoculation

PSYCHOLOGIST DONALD MEICHENBAUM used the principle of cognitive restructuring—changing the way you think—to help people fight stress caused by fear and anxiety. They identified and monitored their negative self-statements. Next they replaced negative statements with coping statements from lists they made up ahead of time. They rehearsed how they would cope with a foreseeable stressful situation, and then they practiced in real life. Periodically his clients returned to get another "inoculation" after their initial training, in order to strengthen the skills that were learned and practiced.

> Inoculate yourself with optimism boosters.

Give yourself "optimism boosters" to inoculate yourself against weight-loss-related pessimism. The tendency to revert to old habits, like overeating, especially in times of stress, is human. Familiarity comforts us. Mothers are familiar with toddlers who, after having been weaned from the bottle want it back again when they are stressed, tired, or sick. Old habits are reassuring when we feel vulnerable and confused.

Self-Reasoning

BE A PROBLEM-SOLVER in the face of difficulty by finding positive solutions and refusing to fall prey to helplessness. For example, perhaps when you are bored, you overeat just for something to do.

When you have identified boredom as the problem, talk yourself through the problem-solving process. For example, you know that boredom leads you to overeat. You might tell yourself, "Sure I feel bored because my friends are all busy tonight. I feel like going for that pint of chocolate ice-cream but I don't want to feel bad about myself afterwards. What do I do to avoid overeating?

Next, identify some alternative solutions to help you cope. As a possibility, you can set the timer for 5 minutes and resolve to refrain from eating until those five minutes are up. By that time most urges to eat will have passed. Another technique is to make plans to go out with a family member, so you won't be in the house concentrating on feeling bored and wanting to eat. The next step is to follow through. Mentally practice the coping statements ahead of time so you will be prepared to put them into practice when actually faced with the situation.

Learning how to cope with difficulties and find solutions keeps us from feeling helplessness and pessimistic. The research indicates that optimists take better care of themselves, live longer, and feel happier. If you are someone who tends to see the glass as half-empty, remember that you can *change your mind* simply by reasoning with yourself.

The Dalai Lama advocates self-reasoning to promote a positive state of mind and to overcome attitudes, thoughts, and emotions that lead to suffering and discontent. Reasoning with yourself leads to a deeper understanding of the problem and tends to put it in a more realistic light. The more you practice replacing negative self-talk with rational coping statements, the more permanent your "cognitive shift" will become.

Fortify yourself with alternatives to fall back upon.

17

A Sample Plan

OBSERVATION IS A POWERFUL LEARNING TOOL. Watching others succeed at something we want to do makes us feel more confident and more motivated to reach our goal. Chris is a good example. She is a "hands-on" person when it comes to her health. She knows her physical and psychological states are intertwined, and respects what her body does for her. She decided to lose a few pounds to lower her risk of heart disease, and feel better about herself in general. She chose a plan that would allow her the freedom to eat and exercise sensibly, with variety.

Sample Journal Entry

CHRIS WROTE OUT THE STEPS she went through, when she first made the decision to lose weight. The journal provides a way for Chris to review the process she went through, and the techniques she used that were modified and refined, as she got further into the process of losing weight. Take a look at the steps that Chris followed on her road to success.

Step One: I will choose an eating plan that includes the foods I really like. It is based on nutritious food choices that include a balance of complex carbohydrates, protein, and lots of fruits and vegetables. I will cut out foods made with white flour and replace them with whole grains. I will eat three meals a day and one snack around 3 or 4 p.m. when I feel my stomach gnawing. When I am not hungry, I will skip the snack. I will drink 8 glasses of water and take a multivitamin each day.

Breakfast Choices:

> French toast made in a non-stick pan with no-sugar preserves or a dollop of yogurt on top.

> Vegetable omelet made with 2 egg whites and one yolk and as many vegetables as I can fit in.

> Low fat cottage cheese with fresh berries.

> Bowl of low-sugar cereal with soy milk.

> Half a bagel with low fat cream cheese and fresh fruit.

> Container of low-fat, low sugar yogurt with fresh fruit.

> Protein soy shake with banana.

Lunch Choices:

> Sliced turkey sandwich on whole wheat with lettuce, tomato, and low-fat mayo

> Small portion of previous night's leftover supper.

> Small can of tuna mixed into a tossed salad with low fat dressing

Slice of low-fat cheese, shredded carrots
and raisins on whole wheat toast.

Egg-salad made with low-fat mayo and
mustard on top of a garden salad.

Veggie burger and oven baked fries.

Supper Choices:

Baked or broiled salmon, tuna, or chicken
with stir-fried or steamed vegetables
and a salad.

Pasta primavera with a large tossed salad.

Vegetarian chili with brown rice.

Pasta all'aglio olio (spaghetti with garlic
and olive oil), and broccoli.

Homemade soup that is low in salt and
fat.

Step Two: I'll make the following entries into my journal every day:

What I ate and drank.

The times I ate and drank.

The place where I ate.

How I felt when I was eating.

What exercise I did during the day.

Situations causing difficulty or stress.

How I coped with difficulties.

What strategies I could use to better cope
next time I face that difficulty.

What I can say to myself to turn my
perceptions from negative to
positive.

Step Three: I'll follow an exercise plan I like.   My
weekly routine will have variety and include all of the
components of exercise that I need. I like change
otherwise I get bored. I also need something that fits
my schedule. Because daily trips to the gym are not
an option for me, this is what I will do:

> Power Yoga 3 mornings a week.
> Total body weight-lifting with light dumb-
>   bells, twice a week in a.m.
> Walk a mile or more every night after
>   dinner.

**Step Four: I'll do special things for myself   to stay
motivated.** The things that were the most msotivating
in the past are:

> 10 minutes of meditation before going to
>   bed.
> Optimistic explanations for upsetting
>   situations.
> Focusing on individual behaviors instead
>   of a long-range weight-loss goals.
> Rewarding myself every week for sticking
>   to my plan.
> Reversing small weight gains right away
> Stop putting myself down for slip-ups
> Making time for favorite activities and
>   people.
> Learning something new everyday.
> Making eating out a celebration of the
>   company not the food.
> Getting regular medical checkups.

Spread Hope Around

MOTIVATIONAL EXPERT MARTIN E. FORD believes that *motivation, skill, biological readiness,* and *a responsive environment* are four ingredients we need to reach our goals. You now have these four ingredients at your disposal. You know how to increase your *motivation* by choosing to think differently in the face of difficulty. You have figured out behavioral *skills* and techniques to support the cognitive changes you've made. You realize that everyone is capable of improving their fitness level, no matter what their *biological* make-up is. Finally, you have a plan to handle the toxic stimuli in your *environment*—including unhealthy foods and psychologically unhealthy people who try to sabotage your efforts.

Weight-loss success depends on making a plan and keeping your eye on the ball. Don't wait for spontaneous motivation, inspiration, or the Tooth Fairy to fall from the sky and do it for you. It takes work, and you have just what it takes to accomplish that work. When you change your mind to change your weight you will feel happier in all areas of your life as you reap the rewards of mental and physical well-being.

Recommended Reading

Bandura, Albert. *Social Foundations of Thought & Action: A Social Cognitive Theory.* Prentice-Hall, 1986.

Bolton, Robert, *People Skills: How to Assert Yourself, Listen to Others and Resolve Conflicts.* Simon & Schuster, 1979.

Csikszentmihalyi, Mihaly, *Finding Flow: The Psychology of Engagement with Everyday Life.* Basic Books, 1997.

Dalai Lama & Cutler, Howard C., *The Art of Happiness: A Handbook for Living.* Riverhead, 1998.

Ellis, Albert, & Robert A. Harper, *A Guide to Rational Living.* Wilshire, 1997.

Ford, Martin E., *Motivating Humans: Goals, Emotions, and Personal Agency Beliefs.* Sage, 1992.

Goleman, Daniel, *Emotional Intelligence: Why It Can Matter More Than IQ.* Bantam, 1995.

Harpaz, Mickey, *The Anti-Diet: How to Eat, Lose, & lLve.* Aitan, 1996.

Hergenhahn, B.R., & Olson, Matthew H., *An Introduction to the Theories of Learning.* Simon & Schuster, 1997.

Hirschmann, Jane R. & Carol H. Munter, *Overcoming Overeating.* Fawcett Columbine, 1988.

Kostas, Georgia, G., *The Balancing Act: Nutrition and Weight Guide.* Arcata Graphics, 1993.

Liebert, Robert M. & Michael D. Spiegler, *Personality: Strategies and Issues*. Brooks/Cole, 1994.

Mautner, Raeleen D., "Cross-cultural explanations of body image disturbance." *International Journal of Eating Disorders,* Sept, 2000.

Mautner, Raeleen D., *9 Made-in-Italy Principles for Living La Dolce Vita.* Sourcebooks, 2002.

Myers, David G., *The Pursuit of Happiness: Discovering the Pathway to Fulfillment, Well-Being, and Enduring Personal Joy.* Avon, 1992.

Potter, Beverly A., *High Performance Goal Setting*. Ronin, 2000.

Schoenfeld, Brad, *Sculpting Her Body Perfect.* Human Kinetics, 1999.

Schoenfeld, Brad, *Look Great Naked: Slim down, Shape Up and Tone Your Trouble Zones in Just 15 Minutes a Day.* Prentice Hall, 2001.

Seligman, Martin E.P., *Helplessness: On Depression, Development and Death.* Freeman, 1975.

Seligman, Martin E.P., *Learned Optimism: How to Change Your Mind and Your Life.* Pocket Books, 1990

Seligman, Martin E.P., *What You Can Change: The Complete Guide to Successful Self-Improvement.* Fawcett Columbine, 1993.

Swenson, Doug, *Power Yoga for Dummies.* Hungry Minds, 2001.

Thomas, Paul R.. (Ed), Institute of Medicine, *Weighing the Options: Criteria for Evaluating Weight-Management Programs.* National Academy, 1995.

Weil, Andrew, *Eating Well for Optimum Health.* Knopf, 2000.

Thompson, J. Kevin (Ed), *Body Image, Eating Disorders, and Obesity: An Integrative Guide for Assessment and Treatment.* American Psychological Association, 1996.

Vedral, Joyce L., *The Fat-Burning Workout.* Warner, 1991.

RONIN Books for Independent Minds